P9-DFZ-030

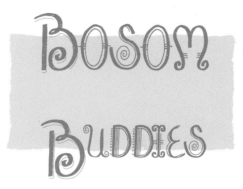

BOSOM BUDDIES

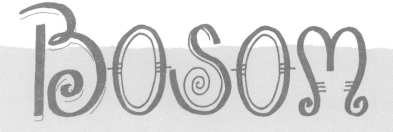

LESSONS AND LAUGHTER
ON BREAST HEALTH AND CANCER

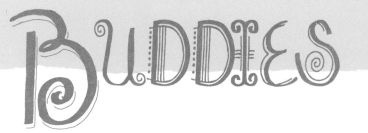

Rosie O'Donnell,
Deborah Axelrod, M.D., F.A.C.S.

with Tracy Chutorian Semler

WARNER BOOKS

A Time Warner Company

If you purchase this book without a cover you should be aware that this book may have been stolen property and reported as "unsold and destroyed" to the publisher. In such case neither the author nor the publisher has received any payment for this "stripped book."

PUBLISHER'S NOTE: In this book the authors are not engaged in rendering medical or other professional services. If an individual is considering changes in his or her health-related practices and regimens, then medical advice or other expert assistance is required, and the services of a competent physician or other professional person should be sought.

All profits from the sale of this book will be distributed as follows:

The National Breast Cancer Coalition (NBCC),
1707 L Street, Suite 1060, Washington, DC 20036 (35%)

The National Alliance of Breast Cancer Organizations (NABCO),
9 East 37th Street, New York, NY 10016 (35%)

SHARE – Self-Help for Women with Breast or Ovarian Cancer,
1501 Broadway, Suite 1720, New York, NY 10036 (20%)

Susan G. Komen Breast Cancer Foundation, Inc.
5005 LBJ Freeway, Suite 370, Dallas, TX 75244 (10%)

Copyright © 1999 by Lucky Charms Entertainment, Inc., and Deborah Axelrod, M.D. All rights reserved.

Warner Books, Inc., 1271 Avenue of the Americas, New York, NY 10020

Visit our Web site at www.twbookmark.com

 A Time Warner Company

Printed in the United States of America

First Printing: November 1999

10 9 8 7 6 5 4 3

LC: 99-65182
ISBN: 0-446-67620-9

Design by Stanley S. Drate/Folio Graphics Co. Inc.
Illustrations by Arlene Frasca
Photography by Lou Manna

To Roseann, Bernice, and Pat—my three mothers
—Rosie O'Donnell

To my family: Noel, Max, Ben, Ann, Murray, and Ruth
—Dr. Deborah Axelrod

*To Nicholas, Drew, and Zachary, my darling
bosom (feeding) buddies*
—Tracy Chutorian Semler

ACKNOWLEDGMENTS

The authors wish to thank the following people for their generous assistance in bringing *Bosom Buddies* to fruition:

Ruth Axelrod, R.N., J.D., and Barbara Ryan, R.N., J.D., Aaronson, Rappaport, Feinstein & Deutsch; Blake Cady, M.D., Women and Infants Hospital of Rhode Island, Providence; Manjeet Chadha, M.D., Marie Frimence, R.N., Ellen Gold, M.D., Josh Gross, M.D., and Bert Petersen, M.D., Beth Israel Medical Center, NYC; Mary Kay Dabney, M.S., St. Luke's–Roosevelt Hospital, NYC; Kristine Dahl, Sean Desmond, and Amanda (Binky) Urban, ICM, NYC; Devra Lee Davis, Ph.D., World Resource Institute, Washington, D.C.; Mary Donovan, J.D., Donovan & Yee, NYC; Stan Drate and staff of Folio Graphics; Judah Folkman, M.D., Harvard Medical School & Children's Hospital, Boston; Colin Fox, Harvey-Jane Kowal, Sharon Krassney, Mari C. Okuda, Anna Maria Piluso, and Jamie Raab, Warner Books; Jeremy Geffen, M.D., Geffen Cancer Center and Research Institute, Vero Beach, Florida; Barry Goldenberg, M.D.; Stan Mack; The National Alliance of Breast Cancer Organizations; Norman King; Larry Norton, M.D., Memorial Sloan-Kettering Cancer Center; Pamela Klein, M.D., National Cancer Institute; Cindy Knauer, R.N., O.C.N.; Kathy Plesser, M.D., Bonnie Reichman, M.D., and Beth Siegel, M.D., St. Vincent's Medical Center, NYC; Noel Raskin, M.D., (for the idea!); David Rose, M.D., Ph.D., D.S.c., American Health Foundation; Linda Secher, Appearance Center Consultants; H. Eric Semler; the staff of the *Rosie O'Donnell Show*; Fran Visco, J.D.; and National Breast Cancer Coalition.

CONTENTS

PREFACE

We can all agree at the outset that there is nothing funny about breast disease, let alone breast cancer.

Why, then, an attempt to blend humor with education about so serious a subject?

Because Rosie, with her gift of giggle, has shown that humor can open the floodgates of curiosity, a willingness to listen, and an eagerness to learn about something that might otherwise be too painful to discuss. Humor helps wipe away fear; it helps lessen anxiety; and it opens both the ears and the spirit. In this receptive mind-set—the mind-set of laughter—women are poised to learn some very important lessons, and to make some very smart decisions.

In short, laughter is the best medicine.

Nowhere was that made more clear than on Rosie's show last October, when she offered free "I Got Squished" T-shirts to women who obtained a screening mammogram—the lifesaving breast X ray that helps detect cancer in its earliest stages. Imagine this: after just one month promoting the subject, laughing about it, schmoozing about it, Rosie's program prompted a staggering 122,457 women to get mammograms! I appeared as a guest on the show and had the great privilege of helping to educate millions of women about the importance of breast disease.

We will never know how many thousands of women were diagnosed with cancers or other abnormalities early enough to lengthen or save their lives. And countless others allayed their deepest fears by finding that they had, in fact, no breast abnormalities at all. A clean bill of health is enormously freeing—but the thousands of women who don't screen their breasts each year never find that out.

As true as it is that there is nothing funny about breast cancer, it is also true that there is nothing hopeless about it—except hopelessness. This book is brimming with examples of how simple information can empower women to protect their breasts and their lives by taking a few steps in self-care: by expanding and improving our dialogue with doctors and other health care providers; by understanding breast anatomy and how it changes over a lifetime; and just by paying attention to our body's signs, so that we can react—and act—on behalf of our own health.

This book represents our many years' experience listening to and learning from women—from Rosie's audience, and from my patients. We try to answer the most-asked questions, address the most-feared topics, and destigmatize the most-held secrets and myths.

We stand poised at the beginning of a new millennium that promises enormous strides in new procedures, new medications, new protocols, and a new understanding about how breast cancer works and how to reduce our risks. Let us seize this critical moment and join the fight against breast cancer, not only to protect ourselves, but our daughters, granddaughters, sisters, friends, and the greater "family" of women—and men—we will never meet, but whose fears and hopes we all share.

BE WELL, GET WELL, AND STAY WELL.

—Deborah Axelrod, M.D.

INTRODUCTION

OK, ladies, listen up . . . this is about the breast, arguably the most famous body part in the history of humankind. The breast, a/k/a titties, tatas, knockers, bosoms, bazoombas, chi chis, Lucy & Ethel—I could go on all day, but I'll stick with boobs.

It's a lifelong odyssey, ours with the breast. We are young, we wonder when we will get them—what will they be like, will they be too flat, too big, too soft, too hard, too round, too pointy, pert or sad, perfectly matched or a bit askew? What about a bra? Is it time? Back from summer vacation, that new girl's shirt had the definite outline of bra in the back. A little scary, a little titillating. All right, here they come—get a training bra. Thwack! The first snap of a bra strap.

We are older, and who knew boobs could be such a delight? Then, for some, come babies and the saga of the boob becomes even more remarkable—milk! And then, well, things can go south, get a bit droopy—like everything else.

They are powerful, these boobs—symbolically and literally they are a force of pleasure, sustenance, motherhood, womanhood, and life itself. They can also be a source of trouble. These days it's hard to find someone whose life has not been touched in some way by breast cancer. A mother, grandmother, sister, aunt, teacher, friend, neighbor—you. My three maternal figures have all gotten it. My mother died of it when I was ten, my best friend Jackie's mother got it and beat it, and my junior high math teacher Pat is battling it now.

Seeing these struggles up close, talking to the women I've met through my show, and grappling with my own fears, I realized that there are so many things I don't know about the boob—and I've got to figure I'm not alone. So, when my doctor, Deborah Axelrod, asked if I would help with this book, I jumped at the chance.

Our mission: demystify the boob. We set out to ask and answer a lot of questions. We talked to many people—some famous, some not so famous. Some doctors, some patients, some survivors—people with answers and observations. We asked questions that are embarrassing, scary, funny, obvious, and obscure—some I never would have thought to ask but am very grateful for the answers. So much to know about the boob!

It seems plain that the more we know, the better equipped we will be to live life together with our boobs instead of in fear of them—and besides, 100 percent of the profits from this book go to breast cancer charities. Many, many thanks to all who have participated in this book, to share their reflections on boobs, bazoombas, titties . . . (there I go again).

—Rosie O'Donnell,
June 1999

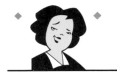

TAKE TWO

See how well you can find the words in this puzzle, and those throughout the book. I can guarantee that these are among the few tests your doctor's *not* going to force you to take.

And although I'm not about to help you find your own boobs, you'll find the answers to the puzzles in the back of the book.

E	L	M	Z	F	H	D	J	F	J	J	M	A	M	M	A	R	I	E	S
M	G	E	V	M	C	A	E	G	S	G	H	B	U	S	T	D	T	W	Q
F	U	W	H	O	P	P	E	R	S	B	R	E	A	S	T	S	I	B	V
N	N	W	B	O	S	O	M	P	E	C	S	G	Y	P	M	R	T	O	H
L	N	G	K	K	R	Y	G	K	H	L	Y	O	D	P	Q	V	S	O	T
B	O	O	B	I	E	S	G	A	Z	O	N	G	A	S	G	V	D	B	K
G	M	G	H	V	T	O	B	G	R	A	P	E	F	R	U	I	T	S	N
J	L	E	Q	O	O	Q	P	H	T	P	U	H	X	K	D	Z	M	S	O
G	M	O	L	Q	O	C	B	S	D	T	I	T	T	I	E	S	D	G	C
L	P	C	B	O	H	R	B	A	Z	O	N	G	A	S	B	N	P	R	K
O	C	R	A	E	N	G	L	J	C	N	V	R	X	P	U	P	B	X	E
P	G	D	H	S	S	S	C	C	L	H	F	C	S	O	G	M	T	O	R
M	X	X	O	I	N	I	C	H	E	S	T	M	M	S	B	R	S	V	S
V	H	E	A	D	L	I	G	H	T	S	O	L	V	R	I	P	K	Y	R
I	R	M	J	D	Y	O	T	Q	X	O	G	D	C	E	T	G	C	T	G
X	I	P	O	R	B	S	H	K	Z	U	K	Y	G	K	E	L	S	A	R
V	Y	P	O	E	H	L	B	A	V	J	U	U	I	N	S	A	G	T	A
I	A	L	Z	A	U	T	B	T	O	R	P	E	D	O	S	N	U	A	C
V	R	U	R	S	R	B	O	U	L	D	E	R	S	H	B	D	J	S	K
E	Q	X	B	S	D	E	C	B	O	M	X	W	F	X	R	S	B	V	T

Find and circle the following words:

BAZONGAS	BREASTS	GLOBES	KNOCKERS	RACK
BAZOOMS	BUGBITES	GRAPEFRUITS	MAMMARIES	TATAS
BOOBIES	BUST	HEADLIGHTS	MELONS	TITS
BOOBS	CHEST	HONKERS	MOUNDS	TITTIES
BOSOM	GAZONGAS	HOOTERS	ORBS	TORPEDOS
BOULDERS	GLANDS	JUGS	PECS	WHOPPERS

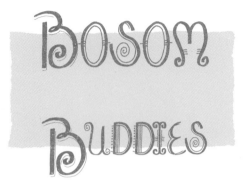

BOSOM BUDDIES

OVERVIEW

~~~~~~

BREAST BUDDIES, BREAST CANCER

BETTY FORD

In August of 1974, seven weeks after my husband was sworn in as president of the United States, a lump was found in my right breast. This came about through an annual checkup at the Bethesda Naval Hospital. At the time of the physical, I was not aware of anything unusual. On returning to the White House, I received a call from the White House physician, Dr. William Lukas. He wanted my husband and me to meet in his office at seven o'clock that evening. He had a breast cancer specialist coming in to examine me. The thought of this was very terrifying. Then our daughter Susan came to me in tears and said, "Oh, Mom, I'm so scared you're going to die." You see, the next day they were scheduling a biopsy followed by surgery, if necessary.

That was how people perceived cancer in those days and there was little discussed about breast cancer. There wasn't a great deal known then. Cancer was a word that was whispered; people did not talk about it in an open way. If somebody had cancer, and particularly breast cancer, it was a topic that people covered up and only whispered behind their hand so no one would hear it. Cancer was such an unknown. So it was a real awakening for the women in the United States to have the wife of the president have breast cancer and speak of it. The realization, "My heavens, if she can have breast cancer, I can, too. It could happen to me also." There was a tremendous reaction. Immediately women wanted to go for breast examinations to find out if they, too, could possibly have breast cancer. People were shocked and yet they became more open about addressing the issue.

Fortunately, they detected my cancer in the early stages and I had a modified radical mastectomy, which involved removal of three lymph nodes. I also underwent chemotherapy for two years, which at that time was somewhat experimental.

The one thing I have found with people who have breast cancer, who've come pretty close to the edge, is that they value each day, and they appreciate life in a new way. For me, it was strengthening of my spiritual being.

◆ WHO SHOULD READ THIS BOOK?

The shorter answer would be to the question "Who should *not* read this book?" The fact is, everyone needs to know about breast cancer. Especially healthy women, who have a tendency to believe that this disease doesn't affect them. I can't tell you the number of patients—healthy, strong women—who eat well, exercise, and take care of themselves in every way, but end up with breast cancer. "How could this happen to me? I'm not a sick person!" they inevitably say. True, there is a lot we can do to catch breast cancer early and often survive it. And we are learning more every day about what we can do to reduce our risks. But we cannot *prevent* breast cancer—*yet*. The self-blame, and the second-guessing about everything you put in your mouth, every aspect of your lifestyle, is pointless. And yet so hard to avoid when facing this disease.

So this book serves a single, vital purpose: to arm *all* women (and men, for that matter), regardless of age and background, with the information and resources needed to beat breast cancer, both physically and emotionally. Because no one is immune to this disease, we must all become educated, armed with information that will allow us to catch cancer early; to use screening tests optimally; to know our bodies when we're healthy so we can recognize worrisome changes; and to understand what puts us at greater risk of getting breast cancer. If needed, we should be able to select the best treatments available around the country; and, if diagnosed with breast cancer, to live a rich life afterward. I can't think of anyone who *doesn't* need this book. I know I do.

◆ WHAT IS BREAST CANCER?

Cancer refers to a group of related diseases that involve out-of-control growth of cells in the body. Normally, healthy cells grow and divide in a regular, set rhythm as they move through their life cycles. With cancer, the growth and division of cells go haywire, with erratic change and proliferation. When these abnormal, cancerous cells group together, they form what's known as a tumor, which penetrates and destroys healthy tissue. When people talk about a cancerous breast lump, or malignant mass, they're referring to a cancerous tumor. In the case of breast cancer, these malignant cells originate in the breast tissue, so the tumor develops somewhere inside the breast. There are two basic cell types of breast cancer, but tumors have many different characteristics that distinguish them from each other. Some are more aggressive than others. We'll talk about many of these characteristics later in this book.

In time, some breast cancers can spread out of the breast to other sites in the body. This is known as metastatic disease. Breast cancer can travel to the lungs, the brain, and the bones, for example. In this case, breast cancer becomes known as the "primary" site—with distant spread of cancer developing afterward. Fortunately, however, with the advent of excellent screening technology, most breast cancers are now caught early, before they have had a chance to spread. This is when breast cancer is most treatable.

Still, breast cancer remains by far the most common cancer among women worldwide, and the leading cause of death in American women aged forty to fifty-nine. In 1999, 175,000 new cases of invasive breast cancer, and 39,900 cases of carcinoma-in-situ (breast cancers limited to the duct) will be diagnosed in the United States. Breast cancer is the third most common cancer in the world.

◆ **WHAT ARE SOME OF THE MAIN TYPES OF BREAST CANCER?**

Most breast cancers fall into a family known as "adenocarcinomas," which means that they originate in the glandular tissue of the breast. Within this category, they go by a variety of scientific-sounding names. For instance: DCIS, or ductal carcinoma-in-situ, the most common form of *noninvasive* breast cancer, is in this family. So is IDC, which stands for infiltrating or invasive ductal carcinoma (it originates in the milk ducts in

FIVE THINGS SCARIER THAN CANCER:

1. Big, ugly spiders

2. The "Snow White" Oscar number with Rob Lowe

3. Any outfit we wore in the '70s

4. If your gynecologist turns out to be Dr. Hannibal Lecter

5. Christopher Walken

the breast (see anatomy, page 26), and then breaks out of that area to invade the breast's fatty tissue. Another relatively common cancer that falls into this category is ILC, for infiltrating or invasive lobular carcinoma—which begins in the milk-producing glands and can invade nearby tissue as well. And finally, a last member of this group is known as LCIS—for lobular carcinoma-in-situ—which is *technically* not a cancer, but can raise the risk of a cancer later in life. I'll talk about each of these types of breast cancer in various places throughout this book.

There are other special subtypes of breast cancer that are associated with a good prognosis. These include (1) "medullary breast cancer," an invasive type of tumor that accounts for about 1 out of 20 cases of breast cancer; (2) "mucinous carcinoma" (also called "colloid cancer"), which, as its name suggests, is created by mucus-producing cancer cells; (3) "papillary" breast cancer, which can be noninvasive or invasive; and (4) "tubular carcinoma," which accounts for approximately 1 out of 50 breast cancer cases and rarely travels to the lymph nodes.

And finally, other relatively rare breast cancer presentations include: (1) Paget's disease, which starts in breast ducts at the level of the nipple and then spreads to the skin of the nipple and areola, where it sometimes appears as a sore or other visible lesion; (2) "inflammatory breast cancer"—an invasive type of breast tumor that accounts for only about 1 out of 100 breast cancer cases; and (3) Phyllodes tumor, which is only rarely malignant and develops in the connective tissue of the breast.

So you can see, a diagnosis of breast cancer doesn't mean just one thing.

◆ Who gets breast cancer?

There are many myths about who gets breast cancer, and what causes it. The fact is, anyone can get breast cancer. It's far more common in women, but men get it, too. Young people get breast cancer; old people get it, too. Rich people get it, and so do the poor. People of all races and ethnicities get breast cancer. Large-breasted women get it; and small-breasted women get it. And despite the many myths about what raises risk, the majority of women have *no identifiable risk factors* and 90 percent have no significant family history of the disease.

Another prevalent myth about breast cancer is that women who live basically healthy lives—who exercise, eat a healthy diet, don't smoke, and don't drink—don't get it. Would that this were true. Unfortunately, while clean living reduces the risk of many cancers and other major diseases, and certainly makes you feel better, it offers no guaranteed protection against breast cancer. No one is immune to this disease.

In the risk chapter of this book, I take you through a variety of risk factors—both genetic (inherent to the individual) and environmental—that seem to increase the risk of breast cancer. But the troubling fact remains that many women with no such risk factors do develop breast cancer, while many women with a whole host of these risk factors do not develop the disease. We still have a great deal to learn.

BREAST CANCER FAIRY TALE #1

GOLDILOCKS

Once there was a girl named Goldilocks. She was called Goldilocks because she bought a beautiful wig during her chemotherapy and always wore it. One day, she decided to go to the Fake Boob Store because she had gotten a double mastectomy and didn't want to throw away her sassy Victoria's Secret bras. She walked in and saw a whole display of mock breasts. A saleswoman walked over and showed Goldilocks a pair.

"What about these, Mademoiselle?"

Goldilocks squeezed them and pronounced: "These are too soft."

"Oui, Mademoiselle," said the saleslady, holding out another pair. "How do you like these knockers?"

"These are too hard," said Goldilocks.

"Pardonnez-moi!" said the saleslady, becoming exasperated. "Those are our two best brands."

Goldilocks noticed a pair lying off to the side. She picked them up and told the saleslady, "These are just right."

"But Mademoiselle, those are cantaloupes! I plan on eating them with my dietetic lunch!"

"I'll give you ten bucks for them!" said Goldilocks, as she tucked them in her bra and skipped merrily off. And they (Goldilocks and the cantaloupes) lived happily ever after.

◆ ◆

◆ WHAT IS THE RISK OF GETTING BREAST CANCER, AND DOES RISK DIFFER FOR DIFFERENT GROUPS OF WOMEN?

To answer your second question first, yes—the risk differs for different groups of women, for some reasons we understand, and others we do not. Take a look at the following statistics for women from different ethnic groups. You'll see that, for instance, the incidence of breast cancer is almost four times higher in Caucasian women than in Native American women.

If you're interested in your risk of getting breast cancer at different ages, see the table on page 10.

> **BREAST CANCER INCIDENCE PER 100,000 WOMEN**
>
> Caucasians: 113.2
> African Americans: 99
> Asian/Pacific Islanders: 71.4
> Hispanics: (people of Hispanic origin can be of any race): 69.3
> Native Americans: 31.9

◆ WHAT'S THE RISK OF DYING OF BREAST CANCER?

People traditionally think of breast cancer as a death sentence, but this is a far cry from the truth. The risk of developing breast cancer is almost five times higher than the risk of dying of it. That's right—there are a lot of people walking around with breast cancer in their past.

However, statistics here are in some ways disturbing. Breast cancer is not an equal opportunity killer. While, as I said earlier, you are much less likely to die of breast cancer than to get it in the first place, there is some worrisome inequity in the statistics here. For example, while Caucasian women are more likely to *get* breast cancer than are African American women, the latter group is still more likely to *die* of the disease. And black women are more than twice as likely to die of breast cancer than are Hispanic and Asian or Pacific Island women. It is possible that African American women may have biologically more aggressive cancers than Caucasian women; for example,

CINDERELLA

Once there was a scullery maid named Cinderella. She desperately wanted to go to the prince's breast cancer benefit. Every year the benefit was held in a beautiful castle and everyone who made a sizable donation was invited. Cinderella couldn't afford to go because she was low on money due to the fact that her insurance didn't cover all of her breast cancer treatment. One night she was crying when her Fairy Godmother appeared.

"Cinderella," said the Fairy Godmother, "I have made a huge donation in your name for breast cancer research and therefore you can go to the ball. I'm giving you my Porsche but I need it back by midnight because I have a hot date with a podiatrist."

Cinderella was overjoyed. "Thank you, Fairy Godmother!"

"Remember," warned the Godmother, "midnight!"

Cinderella went to the ball and fell in love with the prince at first sight. The prince was in love, too, but right before their first kiss the clock struck midnight!

"Oh no! I've got to return the Porsche!"

Cinderella ran out so quickly, one of her fake boobs fell out of her dress.

The prince picked it up and realized Cinderella must be recovering from breast cancer. This made him love her all the more.

He went door to door asking the women of the kingdom if the fake boob belonged to them, but he had no luck. Finally he rang Cinderella's doorbell, but one of her stepsisters answered the door.

"Hey cutie!" said the evil stepsister. "I ain't donating no money to cancer research, but if you want to make out, I'm game."

"No way!" said the horrified prince. "I'm looking for someone who might fit this boob."

At that moment, Cinderella, who was flossing her stepmother's teeth, said, "That's my boob . . . er, knocker . . . er, bazoom . . . er, that's mine!"

"Cinderella," said the lovesick prince. "Stop flossing for a minute. I love you and we shall be married this afternoon!"

"That is so unfair!" said the evil stepsister.

Cinderella gingerly placed the breast inside her bra and applied a little blush and eyeliner. She then ran to the chapel, got married to the prince (her Fairy Godmother and the podiatrist gave her away), and they lived happily ever after.

their tumors are more often "estrogen receptor–negative," which means that the tumors can be harder to control. But this disproportionate percentage of deaths may reflect a wider number of factors, including poorer access to mammography screening and other breast cancer detection tools, less community awareness and education about breast cancer, lower income levels, and other important issues. But whatever the reasons, there is a clear, important problem in need of rectifying. Here are the statistics.

The disturbing statistics about African American women and breast cancer are reflected in similar data for colon and rectal cancers. Black women are also more likely to die of *these* cancers than women of any other racial or ethnic group.

RISK OF DYING FROM BREAST CANCER PER 100,000 WOMEN

Caucasians: 26
African Americans: 31.5
Hispanics (people of Hispanic origin can be of any race): 15.3
Asian/Pacific Islanders: 11.6
Native Americans: 11.7

◆ IS BREAST CANCER PREDOMINANTLY AN OLDER
  WOMAN'S DISEASE?

The incidence of breast cancer increases with age—however, breast cancer is every woman's disease. One-quarter of all women who get breast cancer are under fifty. However, in the African American population, more than one-third of all women with breast cancer are under the age of fifty. Of all breast cancer cases, here is the percentage breakdown by age.

Under thirty: 0.3 percent
Thirty to thirty-nine: 4.8 percent
Forty to forty-nine: 18.1 percent
Fifty to fifty-nine: 18.3 percent
Sixty to sixty-nine: 20.3 percent
Seventy to seventy-nine: 24.2 percent
Over eighty: 14 percent

◆ DOES THE RISK OF BREAST CANCER VARY BY
  INCOME LEVEL?

Breast cancer patients in the lower income bracket have a 9 percent lower five-year survival rate than women of higher income. And lower-income African American women are three times more likely than higher-income African American women to be diagnosed at an advanced stage of breast cancer. Clearly, poverty is an important determining factor in terms of a woman's chance of surviving breast cancer.

◆ IS BREAST CANCER BEING CAUGHT EARLIER
  THESE DAYS?

Yes—cancers are being caught earlier, when they are smaller; and also, women diagnosed with early breast cancer are less likely to be "lymph node positive"—meaning that these days, when the cancer is found, it's less likely than in days past to have spread to the lymph nodes under that armpit. The tool most responsible for the hopeful trend toward catching earlier cancers is the mammogram, or breast X ray. Generally, women who have information about and access to this type of screening have a better chance at early detection and long-term survival. I'll talk a lot about this excellent tool, which is used both for screening and for diagnosis, throughout this book.

However, the trend to earlier diagnosis is not equal among women of different racial backgrounds. For example, among Caucasian women, 62 percent of breast cancers are caught when they are still confined to the breast; 29 percent are found when they have spread only to the lymph nodes under the arm; and 6 percent are found when they have spread to distant sites. Among African American women, only 50 percent of breast cancers are caught when they are still confined to the breast; 35 percent are found when they have spread to the underarm lymph nodes; and 9 percent are detected at distant sites. In sum, African American women are more likely to be diagnosed with more advanced breast cancer. And this is very disturbing, because when cancers are caught earlier, they are easier to treat—and the prognosis is generally better.

Just take a look at these five-year survival rates:

For Caucasian women with localized cancer—that is, cancer contained in the breast—the five-year survival rate is an impressive 98 percent. For African American women, it's just 89 percent. For breast cancer that has spread "regionally"—that is, to the underarm lymph nodes—the five-year survival rate is 78 percent among Caucasian women, but just 62 percent among African American women. And finally, when you compare the five-year survival rates for women with *distant* disease—that is, breast cancer that has spread to distant sites in the body—the discrepancy between the races continues to be quite disturbing: a 23 percent survival rate for Caucasian women, and just 14 percent for African American women.

◆ ARE FEWER PEOPLE DYING OF BREAST CANCER THESE DAYS?

Yes, and no. Between 1990 and 1995, the most recent available data, breast cancer mortality rates dropped 1.7 percent per year. But again, the good news has not been evenly distributed.

SOME BREAST CANCER TV EPISODES
THAT NEVER MADE IT:

HAPPY DAYS—The Fonz gets male breast cancer and is bummed out because he has a date with Pinky Tuscadero. The day is saved when Joanie pronounces: "Don't worry, Fonz . . . Pinky has enough breast for both of you!"

LAVERNE AND SHIRLEY—Laverne thinks she found a lump in her breast but is relieved when Squiggy discovers that a Junior Mint fell down her bra.

THREE'S COMPANY—Mr. Furley walks in on the gang doing a breast self-exam, and threatens to evict them unless one of them has a lump. In a desperate bid to save the apartment, Jack creates a lump out of a biscuit. Hilarity ensues when Chrissy eats the biscuit by mistake.

GILLIGAN'S ISLAND—Ginger fakes breast cancer in order to get off the island. The Professor agrees to give her a mammogram using two coconuts and bamboo shoots. Ginger's ruse is figured out when the coconuts register not only an absence of cancer, but silicone breasts to boot. Ginger decides to stay and Mary Ann makes a banana cream pie.

THE BRADY BUNCH—Alice goes for a mammogram but Cindy doesn't understand and tells Mr. Brady that Alice left because of a "telegram." The Bradys think Alice must have quit because she had a family emergency and they temporarily hire Jan to replace Alice. In the end, Alice comes home with a clean bill of health, and the Bradys decide to keep Jan on as a maid, but cut her salary.

I LOVE LUCY—The Ricardos and the Mertzes decide to switch roles for a week, forcing Ricky and Fred to get mammograms. Lucy doesn't want the female technician flirting with Ricky, so she and Ethel dress up in white lab coats and try to perform the mammogram themselves! After a locksmith has to pry Lucy from the mammography machine, Ricky declares she has some " 'splainin' to do!"

The decrease was greater among Caucasian women and younger women—most likely thanks to aggressive screening mammography and so-called adjuvant or additional treatments like cancer-fighting drugs.

When you look back a few more years, you'll find some odd-looking statistics about breast cancer incidence: for instance, between 1982 and 1987, the rate of breast cancer *increased* 4 percent per year. Since then, it has remained fairly constant. How could the incidence rates of such a major disease increase for a few years and then suddenly begin to decrease and hold steady? Many researchers believe that the increase in breast cancer screening during the 1980s helped boost the number of breast cancers that were *diagnosed*—thereby creating an artificial increase in the incidence rates. Probably, there were no more new cancers during this period—just more being caught. We need more studies to help clarify if, and why, breast cancer rates may be changing.

◆ WHAT COUNTRIES HAVE THE MOST BREAST CANCER?

The United States has the dubious distinction of leading the world in breast cancer incidence. And in general, the incidence of breast cancer is high in all developed countries, especially in North America, Australia, temperate South America, and northern and western Europe. The notable *exception* to this developed country trend, however, is Japan. Why is there significantly *less* breast cancer in Japan? If we knew the answer for sure, we might have a powerful clue as to how to reduce the incidence everywhere else in the world. Unfortunately, we are left to guess, but there are some leading theories among researchers. One hypothesis centers around diet. Japanese women tend to eat significantly less fat than American women do, and they also eat a relatively large quantity of estrogenic plant-based foods, like soy. I will talk about soy, its potential benefits and risks, later in this book. But in simple terms, soy and other plant-based estrogenic foods may—I repeat *may*—offer a certain degree of protection against breast cancer. As for the low-fat diet, this is another topic I will address several times throughout this book. There is a prominent belief that a low-fat diet promotes lower estrogen levels in the body, thereby reducing the risk of breast cancer. In fact, the ratio of fats in the Japanese diet has been used as a model for a number of American studies looking into the possibility that lowered fat intake might reduce the risk of breast cancer. The theory is that American women may be hurting themselves in two ways at once. When you eat a high-fat diet, as American women do, you tend to displace fiber in the diet as well (think about it: if you're eating eggs and bacon for breakfast, you usually aren't eating cereal and berries). This relative lack of fiber in the American diet may also play a role in promoting breast cancer. The jury is still out on this question. But it continues to interest many scientists around the world, and we hope to have more definitive answers on the subject in the coming years. The bottom line is, no firm data yet exists to show a clear relationship between diet and the risk of breast cancer.

WHERE IN THE WORLD IS BREAST CANCER LEAST COMMON?

Breast cancer rates tend to be low in most of Asia and in sub-Saharan Africa—with the exception of South Africa. The lowest incidence of breast cancer is in China, where only 11.8 out of 100,000 women get the disease. Compare that to 87 out of 100,000 women in the United States, and you get an idea of how major the difference is. Why is China's rate so low? Again, there are no definitive answers, but there are theories. It's not likely to be due to inherited genetic factors, as there is only slight variation in the rate of inheritable breast cancer throughout the world. It's more likely to be environmental—that is, related to diet, or pesticide exposure, or chemicals from industrialization.

When you look at the world as a whole, however, the picture isn't cheerful: the overall incidence of breast cancer is climbing 0.5 percent annually in most places. At this rate, we'll see 1.35 *million* new cancers in the year 2010. And it has been observed that the incidence rates are climbing the most in areas with the lowest previous rates, and in areas with rapid economic/industrial growth. For instance, the rate of increase in China may be as high as 5 percent per year.

I'VE HEARD THAT BREAST CANCER RATES CAN CHANGE WHEN YOU MOVE FROM ONE COUNTRY TO ANOTHER. IS THIS TRUE?

Yes, especially among women who migrate at a young age. And this happens to be one of the important pieces of information that leads researchers to believe that some aspect(s) of the environment is a powerful factor in determining breast cancer risk. For instance, there is some very well-known data about Japanese women moving from Japan to the United States. It appears that these women have relatively low rates of breast cancer in Japan, and then their rates climb significantly when they reach the United States. The increase in risk is especially pronounced among first-, second-, and third generation migrants. Why? Could it be the change in diet? A change in weight? A change in chemicals in the air? A change in pesticides in foods? Postponed childbearing? All of the above? There is a great deal of interest in what makes for changes in the risk of breast and other cancers with migration from place to place. But the data does seem to underscore the fact that a genetic predisposition probably plays a smaller role than environment in promoting such changes in risk—or at least that environmental changes play a major part in promoting risky hormonal effects and triggering cancer genes.

TOP 40 COUNTDOWN

Here are the most-requested songs
by breast cancer patients:

40. "Another One Bites the Bust"

39. "Bust in the Wind"

38. "Boobie Nights"

37. "The Breast Thing That Ever Happened to Me"

36. "One Bad Booby (Don't Spoil the Whole Bunch)"

35. "Summer in the Titty"

34. "Titty Titty Bang Bang"

33. "Rack in the USSR"

32. "Knocker Three Times"

31. "Rack the Knife"

30. "Super-chemotherapeutic-expialidocious"

29. "Brand New Chemo"

28. "Bustghosters"

27. "I Lost My Boob in San Francisco"

26. "Get Down (Boobie Oobie Oobie)"

25. "Jugs the Two of Us"

24. "Breast of Burden"

23. "Love to Love You Booby"

22. "You're 44D (You're Beautiful, and You're Mine)"

21. "You Take My Breast Away"

20. "One Less Boob to Cancer"

19. "This Gland Is Your Gland"

18. "Giving You the Breast That I Got"

17. "Na, Na, Hey, Hey, Good Biopsy"

16. "Mammo Told Me Not to Come"

15. "Rack around the Clock"

14. "Thanks for the Mammaries"

13. "My Girls"

12. "Obla-Di, Obla-Da (Don't Need No Bra)"

11. "I Wanna Hold Your Gland"

10. "Gland on the Run"

9. "Thank God I'm a Country Boob"

8. "X Ray of Light"

7. "It Only Takes a Chemoment"

6. "Deep in the Heart of Pecs-es"

5. "Chemover Beethoven"

4. "Save the Breast for Last"

3. "Chesterday"

2. "My Booby Lies Over the Ocean"

**And the number one most-requested song
by breast cancer patients is . . .**

1. "Shake Your Booby"

◆ ◆

◆ IS IT TRUE THAT MEN CAN GET BREAST CANCER?

Yes. Male breast cancer accounts for less than 1 percent of all breast cancers, with about 1,300 new cases and 400 deaths expected in the U.S. in 1999. Jewish and African American men are at greater risk than others.

The following health problems have been associated with an increased risk of breast cancer in men—but certainly do not *cause* breast cancer.

- mumps orchitis, a testicular infection associated with the mumps
- testicular tumors
- Klinefelter's syndrome—an inherited chromosomal/hormonal problem
- undescended testicles
- exposure to ionizing radiation (also a risk factor for women)
- liver disease
- genetics—such as carrying a mutation in the gene known as BRCA2
- occupational exposure to heat, possibly because of its impact on testicular function

Because men are not routinely screened with mammography (breast X rays), they usually present with some kind of visible or palpable sign—such as a lump in the breast area, an inverted nipple, or bloody discharge.

The most troubling feature of breast cancer in men is that diagnosis is often delayed, mostly because no one suspects the disease, and partly because there is no recommended routine screening. As a result, the average age at diagnosis is sixty-four years—older than in women. And because men's breast cancer is often close to the chest wall, or involves the nipple, it's harder to use breast-conserving surgery (lumpectomy) in men. So mastectomies, or removal of the entire breast, are more common in men these days than in women. Men are likely to develop cancers that are "estrogen receptor–positive," which means that men often receive hormonal treatment with the drug tamoxifen (discussed in more detail on page 168).

Men with a strong family history of breast cancer—that is, a mother or sister with the disease—should talk to their doctor about genetic counseling (more on pages 84 and 105), and about developing some type of regular screening program. Men can carry the so-called BRCA genes for breast cancer, and if they do, they're at increased risk not only for breast cancer, but for cancers of the colon and prostate as well. So vigilant screening for these other cancers is important as well.

Many men—including as many as two-thirds of adolescent boys for a short period of time—have a condition known as gynecomastia, which means female-like breasts—and this condition is *benign*. There are several causes of gynecomastia, including the use of recreational drugs such as marijuana, LSD, and heroin, alcohol, and common prescription drugs such as trycyclic antidepressants, digitoxin (Lanoxin), and cimetidine (Tagamet), among others. For years, people thought that gynecomastia was a precancerous condition, and doctors advocated "subcutaneous mastectomies"—that is, surgical removal of the inside of the breast—to prevent cancer. This is not indicated for medical reasons.

◆ WHAT'S THE LATEST TREND IN BREAST CANCER CARE?

The trend is less invasive, less invasive, less invasive. In the past, major mutilating surgery for breast cancer was common. Today, whether testing tissue to see if it's cancerous or operating on known cancerous tumors, the approach is to get the cancer out with as little manipulation and mutilation as possible. So needle biopsies to remove cells from the breast are gradually replacing more extensive surgical excisions; and when appropriate, lumpectomy (removal of the lump and some normal surrounding tissue) is gradually replacing mastectomy (removal of the entire breast). Between 1983 and 1991, for example, the use of lumpectomy increased from 16 percent to 37 percent while the use of mastectomy declined from 75 percent to 58 percent. In 1994, 43 percent of women had lumpectomy, and 51 percent had radical mastectomy. Less invasive procedures are proving to be equally effective, with less trauma to the bodies and minds of women with breast cancer.

A COUPLA WHITE BOOBS
SITTIN' AROUND TALKING

HAPPY: Hey, what's with you? You look like you're tingling all over.

LUMPY: I am. I've been anesthetized.

HAPPY : Been seeing that doctor again?

LUMPY : Yeah, he's my main squeeze.

HAPPY : He was all over me, too, ya know.

LUMPY : Guess what—he's taking me out tonight!

HAPPY : I thought we were gonna bounce around together.

LUMPY : Sorry, he's just taking me. And I gotta tell you, I'm not coming back.

HAPPY : What?

LUMPY : I heard him say he's interested in a permanent arrangement.

HAPPY : What, are you gonna leave me hanging?

LUMPY : Yup, I'm leaving you flat.

HAPPY : I always knew you'd end up with a doctor.

LUMPY : Bye bye, friend.

HAPPY : Bye . . . and remember . . .

LUMPY : Yes?

HAPPY : We'll always be bosom buddies!

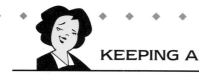

KEEPING ABREAST OF THE PROBLEM

Had enough doctor stuff? Time for a word search. Find these, have fun.

Y	A	C	K	C	K	F	P	W	X	K	O	C	T	B	Y
C	T	Q	N	M	D	X	X	O	W	Y	K	X	R	J	S
R	N	O	W	W	R	R	K	A	L	N	A	P	A	J	A
C	L	S	N	E	G	O	R	T	S	E	O	T	Y	H	P
F	Y	S	R	C	B	W	E	J	J	U	G	H	A	T	K
D	A	P	N	E	G	O	R	T	S	E	G	X	Y	W	O
I	N	B	P	L	O	N	G	I	S	L	A	N	D	L	L
R	W	V	T	H	S	W	L	A	V	F	G	O	L	H	V
N	U	O	L	U	J	I	R	M	W	F	R	C	J	A	C
R	T	A	F	Y	R	A	T	E	I	D	U	H	G	L	K
Q	A	R	S	L	F	F	I	N	L	A	N	D	I	N	W
O	S	E	D	I	C	I	T	S	E	P	F	W	N	D	O
K	K	M	E	F	N	K	M	Z	X	Q	G	I	E	I	M
O	T	Z	W	T	O	E	Y	L	N	K	U	F	B	W	E
Z	Z	X	H	E	I	G	O	U	J	W	Y	O	T	E	N
R	M	O	M	E	N	J	K	I	O	P	P	Y	O	S	R

Find and circle the following words:

DIETARY FAT	JAPAN	PHYTOESTROGENS
ESTROGEN	LONG ISLAND	SOY
FIBER	MEN	WOMEN
FINLAND	PESTICIDES	

1

BOSOM BUDDIES:
Breast Health and Anatomy

PEGGY FLEMING

I noticed my breast lump while looking at my body in the mirror. I was thinking how fit and athletic I was and what good shape I was in. My whole life had been dedicated to healthiness and fitness. It was very difficult, as an athlete, to come to terms with something unhealthy in my body. The fact is, you have to pay attention to yourself and your body. You know your own body better than even your doctor does. And cancer can happen to anyone, no matter how well you take care of yourself.

◆ WHAT'S A NORMAL, HEALTHY BREAST?

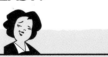

A "normal, healthy breast" comes in many different shapes, sizes, and colors. In fact, I'm not a big fan of the word "normal," as there is such great variability in what's "normal," as well as what's healthy. Normal for you may be quite different from

A healthy breast isn't codependent on its partner.

what it is for other women; and, for that matter, "normal" changes throughout your life cycle, as the breast goes through a wide variety of changes I'll discuss in this chapter. For instance, before you reach puberty and begin menstruating, your breasts tend to be quite smooth inside and out; afterward, with the dramatic shift in hormones within your body, the breasts begin to develop greater texture. With texture can come concerns—suspicious lumps and other nodules that may worry you—but that are most often perfectly harmless. (I'll talk about the kinds of breast changes to worry about later in this chapter.) The bottom line is that big breasts can be healthy and normal; tiny breasts can be healthy and normal; loose, sagging breasts can be healthy and normal; and firm, perky breasts can be healthy and normal. Breasts that are different in size can be healthy and normal (in fact, few women have breasts exactly the same size, and when I see a perfectly matched pair in my office, I always look for the implant scars!). We come in a wide variety of packages. The most important idea to cling to is that you must never fall prey to the billion-dollar advertising campaigns that try to tell you what "normal" breasts look like— usually hard-as-rocks and practically pointing to the ceiling—with lots of cleavage and a golden tan. Sure, the image is an attractive one—but attractive, healthy, and normal come in many other guises as well.

◆ WHAT ARE SOME NORMAL VARIATIONS ON THE EXTERIOR OF THE BREAST?

Let's start with the breast skin. Naturally, depending on what color your overall body skin is, the skin of your breasts will differ. However, no matter what your skin color, the breasts tend to be a little lighter than the rest

Teeth marks.

of your skin—partly because of a relative lack of sun exposure. While some women have extremely smooth and almost hairless breasts, others have fine or even coarse hair on the breasts. The nipple of the breast is usually relatively dark—pinkish or brownish—and protrudes slightly (I'll talk about inverted nipples a bit later). The nipple is surrounded by the areola, a ring of slightly lighter-colored skin than the nipple itself. This area often darkens during pregnancy and breast-feeding (lactation). Often, there are little pimple-like bumps on the areola; these are known as "Montgomery gland tubercles," and they are a cross between sweat glands and breast glands. They sometimes

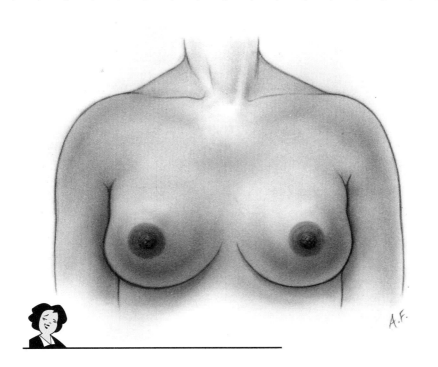

Artist's rendering of my actual breasts.

secrete a watery substance around the time of breast-feeding and pregnancy. Some women worry about these glands—especially if they are increasing in number—and think they are early tumors. But they are perfectly normal, and if you have twice as many as your sister, there's nothing wrong with you—or with her.

The nipple can be very sensitive, as it contains many nerve endings.

◆ SO WHAT SHOULD THE INSIDE OF MY BREASTS BE LIKE?

The picture that follows shows the inside of a healthy breast, which you'll see is a very busy workplace.

Internal Breast Anatomy Side View

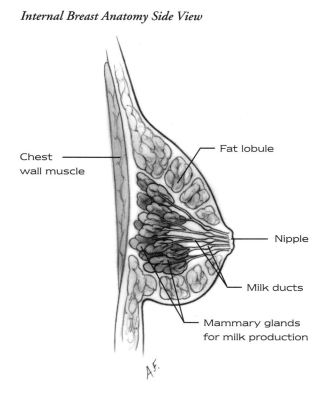

Chest
wall muscle

Fat lobule

Nipple

Milk ducts

Mammary glands
for milk production

Let's go through the various parts of the breast and what they do. Starting right behind the nipple are the biggest tubes inside the breast, called ducts. These ducts are where the milk flows when you breast-feed. Behind the ducts, moving farther back into the breast, are the ductules—smaller tubes that feed into the larger ducts. (Believe it or not, there are twelve to fifteen major duct systems in the breast—it's a complex organ.) Behind the ductules are the lobules. The very smallest of the ducts, farthest away from the nipples and deep in the breast, are the so-called terminal duct lobular units, or TDLU. This happens to be the most susceptible part of the breast to cancer. You can think of the lobules as the factories that produce the breast milk before it is carried through the duct system. The lobules are surrounded by supporting or fibrous tissue, fatty tissue, blood vessels, lymphatic tissue, and nerves. At certain ages, you'll find more or less of this material in the breast. For

Where Problems Occur in the Breast

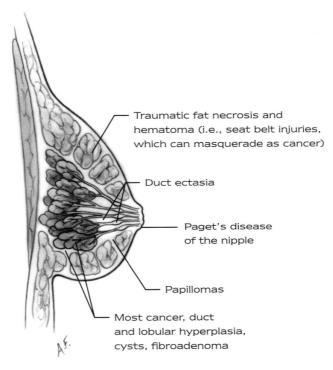

Traumatic fat necrosis and
hematoma (i.e., seat belt injuries,
which can masquerade as cancer)

Duct ectasia

Paget's disease
of the nipple

Papillomas

Most cancer, duct
and lobular hyperplasia,
cysts, fibroadenoma

instance, younger women have a higher ratio of breast cells and
fibrous tissue—and less fat in the breasts. Older women tend
to have the opposite, with more fat, fewer breast cells, and less
fibrous tissue. This is one reason why younger women's breasts
often appear firmer than older women's breasts, and why mammograms are sometimes tougher to read in younger women
(the breast tissue shows up as very dense). Other reasons for the
difference include the strength of the underlying chest muscle,
and the tone of the skin of the breasts.

Throughout the breast you have many little lymph channels, which lead to the lymph nodes under the arm and along
the breastbone. These channels drain the breast of fluid, including waste fluid. On the negative side, this is one of the
means by which cancer cells can travel out of the breast and
into the lymph nodes. The lymph nodes extend from under the
arms into the neck area, and create a rich network with each

other in several areas in the upper body. Later in this book, I'll talk about the importance of checking the lymph nodes for cancer spread in certain cases.

Underneath the breasts lie the chest muscles; and these muscles, in turn, rest on the ribs. Extremely thin women may feel what they believe to be hard lumps in the breast, which actually turn out to be rib bone—particularly between the two breasts, where there is the least overall tissue.

Just to give you an idea of where in the breast various common problems occur, I've created a picture of the internal anatomy of the breast—tagged for various disease processes (see page 27).

It helps a great deal to become educated about the anatomy of your breasts and to be familiar with how different parts of your breasts look and feel. The more you know about your breasts when they are in a baseline "normal" state, the better able you will be to detect new abnormalities *for you*. But no matter what, as I'll discuss later in this chapter, if you're worried about something new or different you feel in your breast, don't try to diagnose it yourself, and don't doubt yourself. Tell your doctor.

◆ SHOULD I WORRY ABOUT "INVERTED NIPPLES"?

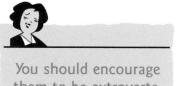

Here is a guiding principle about what should *not* worry you: if it's a long-standing condition that has not changed, it is usually fine. As a breast surgeon, I often don't see women until they have reached midlife—so I haven't had the benefit of seeing their breasts develop

> You should encourage them to be extroverts. Shyness is so often painful.

over a lifetime. For this reason, I take women's reports about their own bodies very seriously. For instance, consider the case of inverted nipples. With inverted nipples, the tip of the nipple does not stick out—it goes inward, into the areolar area.

If a woman tells me that her nipples have been like this her whole life, then I generally don't worry—because inverted nipples are a perfectly normal and healthy variation. Or, if she tells me that her nipples have a tendency to move in and out—which is also common—I usually won't worry. On the other hand, if a woman comes to me and says that her nipple has *recently become inverted*, but used to stick out all of the time—this would raise a red flag. Why? Because a cancer may be pulling on the ligaments, which in turn may be pulling the nipple in. Also, breast surgery can cause benign nipple inversion. Or, perhaps there is another, separate benign condition (i.e., benign inflammation) tugging on the nipple. In any case, further examination may be necessary.

◆ WHAT ARE SOME OTHER VARIATIONS ON "NORMAL" BREASTS THAT I SHOULD *NOT* WORRY ABOUT?

1. Extra nipples, also known as polythelia: About 1 out of every 100 people (men and women) has more than two nipples. They do not necessarily appear on the breast site—they can appear anywhere from the armpits to the groin. This

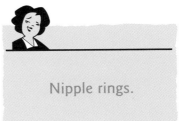

Nipple rings.

condition is also called "accessory nipples"—although the extra nipples are sometimes much more than accessories, as some of them actually can function. For instance, women may be able to breast-feed from an extra nipple. In other cases, you might not even realize you *have* an extra nipple—you just assume all your life that you have a protruding mole. The nipple might be more noticeable if it is attached to extra breast tissue, as well—but this is not always the case.

2. Extra breast tissue, known as polymastia: This is another variation on normal breasts. Some women have extra breast tissue, or what appears to be a full extra breast, somewhere between the usual breast location and the armpit or as low down as the groin. Extra breast tissue can appear with or without an extra nipple, as described above. Extra breast tissue is subject to the same range of changes and problems as

YOU AND YOUR BREASTS QUIZ

1) Do you have a close relationship with your breasts?

   a) Close enough to have given them each their own nickname.
   b) We used to be close, but it seems time has caused us to drift apart.
   c) I haven't seen or spoken to them in years.

2) What do you do to show your breasts that you love them?

   a) Regular doctor appointments, monthly self-exam, and then I take them out for ice cream.
   b) I visit the doctor yearly, and avoid looking at Victoria's Secret catalogues so they won't feel bad about themselves.
   c) What do they ever do to show that they love me?

3) When it's time to have the doctor examine your breasts, you . . .

   a) Rip off your shirt and yell, "How do they look?"
   b) Get a little nervous, but suck it up anyway.
   c) Request that you be put under general anesthesia first.

4) When someone reminds you that smoking and an unhealthy diet both contribute to all types of cancer, you . . .

   a) Smile knowingly because you don't smoke and you eat your veggies.
   b) Promise yourself you won't start smoking, but also add to your will that you would like to be buried with several boxes of Duncan Hines brownie mix.
   c) Think "Great, I'm doomed," and then wonder if it's possible to roll and smoke a cheeseburger.

5) You think you can't get breast cancer because . . .

   a) I don't think that, but I'm doing everything I can to not let it happen, or to catch it early if it does.
   b) Nobody in my family ever had it, and I'm in decent health.
   c) I'm really, really way too busy right now.

6) If you found a lump in your breast, what would you do?

   a) Call my doctor immediately.
   b) Pray that it was a pimple, but if it didn't go away in a day or so, call the doctor.
   c) Think "Great, I'm doomed," and then max out all your credit cards.

7) If you were to compare your breasts' personalities to the personalities of a celebrity's breasts, who would you choose?

   a) Peggy Fleming—the breasts of a survivor.
   b) Pamela Anderson—smart enough to have those implants removed.

   c) That secretary from *The Beverly Hillbillies*—well, at least I'm being honest.

8) If you and your breasts had a TV show, what would it be called?

   a) *Party of Three*—a touching drama about closeness and understanding among loved ones.

   b) *Three's Company*—a funny farce about three living together with all kinds of wacky misunderstandings and pratfalls.

   c) *Rescue 911-36B*—a scary reality-based program about what can happen when you don't keep an eye on your boobs.

9) If your boobs could talk to you, what would they say?

   a) Thank you, thank you, thank you!

   b) We've fallen and we can't get up.

   c) Uh, nice to meet you . . . what was your name again?

10) In five years, where do you see your relationship with your breasts going?

   a) Strong and healthy as ever.

   b) Hopefully improving, appreciating each other more.

   c) For the love of God, I will give you anything if you just stop asking questions about my breasts. I really, really don't want to talk about it, let alone with a complete stranger. Please, please let it be over.

SCORING

For every question you answered with an "a," give yourself two points.

For every question you answered with a "b," give yourself one point.

For every question you answered with a "c," give yourself zero points.

TOTALS

15–20 points—You're a "Best Breast Baby." You know your body and what you need to do to take care of it, especially "the twins." Keep it up, girlfriend!

8–14 points—You've got "Middle of the Road Mammaries." You know your breast-care basics, but you could be doing more for yourself. Take some tips from a friend who's a "Best Breast Baby," and you too could be in the pink!

0–7 points—You're being a "First Class Boob." You're ignoring precious assets that're right under your nose (if you're lucky). Keep it up, and someday, your breasts just might leave you. It's not too late to turn it around, though. Have some pride, get to know 'em, and you just might be able to rekindle the playful and supportive relationship you thought you'd lost.

any other breast: it can become tender before menstruation, it can develop breast cancer, it can lactate (produce milk for breast-feeding), and so on. Some women find that their extra breast tissue appears for the first time after pregnancy, as a result of changing levels of estrogen. The extra breast tissue may then recede after delivery, only to recur with a subsequent pregnancy. Other women have an extra breast all the time. While this is usually a normal condition, it can be extremely upsetting to many women, who are bothered either by the unsightly appearance of an extra breast or by the constant worry that the lump is a tumor in and of itself, and not a separate breast. In other cases, if the extra breast tissue is especially firm or nodular, there may be a malignant process going on, so it's important to be checked by your doctor. In extreme cases, this can appear like a mound the size of a grapefruit under the arm. Even if the tissue is found to be normal, however, if you find an extra breast or mound of breast tissue especially upsetting, and it is hindering your lifestyle in some meaningful way—(e.g., stopping you from wearing sleeveless shirts or bathing suits, or otherwise making you dislike and hide your body from others), you might want to consider having it removed. A plastic surgeon would usually be the one to do the job.

3. Stretch marks: These are pink, white, or silvery lines on the breast, usually slightly indented. Not every woman has stretch marks on her breasts, but many do. They are associated with rapid growth of the breasts during adolescence, and also with dramatic weight gain or loss. They are normal and not an indication of any disease process.

4. Premature or delayed breast development: Girls who develop breasts before age eight and without other signs of puberty (such as underarm or pubic hair) are considered to have *premature* or early breast development. On the other side of the coin, young women who develop breasts after the age of fourteen are considered to have *delayed* or late breast development. Both cases are usually normal, but it's wise to have a doctor check it out. You may need to have certain hormone levels

checked, to be sure that there is no underlying hormonal abnormality causing the atypical breast development.

5. Leaking breasts during pregnancy and/or breast-feeding:
The breasts go through a great deal of change during pregnancy and lactation, and a milky discharge at this time is not
uncommon. Mention it to your doctor to be on the safe side,
but usually this is no cause for alarm. In fact, milky discharge
can occur even up to two years after breast-feeding, as it takes
your breasts quite some time to return to their prefeeding "resting state." See a later question for a discussion of when nipple
discharge is worrisome.

There are many other variations on normal breasts—I
could take up a whole book discussing them. The important
thing is if anything about your breasts worries or frightens you,
talk to your doctor about it. New changes, as I said before, are
more worrisome than conditions or appearances that have been
there for many years. But you shouldn't be the one to decide
what's worrisome and what isn't. Always seek your doctor's input and trust your judgment if something seems awry.

◆ WHAT CHANGES SHOULD I EXPECT IN MY BREASTS DURING PREGNANCY AND BREAST-FEEDING?

During pregnancy and breast-feeding, there is a proliferation of cells in
the breasts. You will develop more
ducts, more lobules, and your breasts
will start to enlarge and become
plump with fluid rich in protein.
This is all in preparation for lacta-

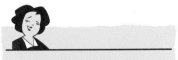

They'll get big . . . and
then a kid will suck
on them.

tion or breast-feeding. The blood flow to your breasts at the end
of pregnancy increases a startling 180 percent, and the breasts
can double in weight at this time. Your nipples and areolar area
may darken during pregnancy and breast-feeding, as well.

Later, after you stop breast-feeding, your breasts may take
as long as two years to return to their "resting state"—that is,
their condition before you became pregnant. Sometimes, there

are permanent visible changes in the breast—such as stretch marks (see page 32), or a bit of sagging or shape change to the breast. Remember, while the breasts become fully developed at about age twenty, they start to show changes associated with age at about age forty. So if you have children in your mid-to-late thirties or later, as is increasingly common, you may see changes in your breasts that are related *both* to age and to the biological shifts of pregnancy and lactation.

◆ WHEN SHOULD I WORRY ABOUT NIPPLE DISCHARGE?

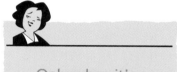

Only when it's a dishonorable discharge.

I tend to worry about nipple discharge when it is spontaneous. By "spontaneous" I mean that the discharge appears when you are *not* touching or squeezing your nipples—e.g., you might just wake up and find it on your nightgown, or discover it in your bra during the day. Many women can elicit some type of discharge from the nipples by squeezing them—but this is rarely an indication of a problem.

Nipple discharge comes in many different colors and consistencies. It may be milky and whitish; creamy; watery and clear; yellow (serous); pink; red (bloody); or it can be multicolored, or greenish. As a rule, green is good, as green discharge often indicates "normal" fibrocystic changes in the breast. In addition, very often you'll find that discharge is multicolored and comes from different openings in the nipple, and this is usually fine as well. A milky discharge during pregnancy or breast-feeding is not worrisome—and can also result from taking certain psychotropic medications, from thyroid disorders, or from oral contraceptive use. But if you have a milky discharge (called galactorrhea) without such an explanation, I recommend a workup to make sure there is no underlying hormonal problem or trouble with the pituitary gland—such as a prolactinoma (a tumor producing the hormone responsible for making milk).

A yellow, pink, red, or clear discharge requires a workup by your doctor. In addition, a discharge associated with a mass also requires medical attention.

Many doctors do a "guaiac" test of the fluid to see if it is bloody. A "smear" test of the cells (on a slide) may also be performed to see if they are benign or cancerous. This is not a definitive test, but if the results are positive—that is, if cancer shows up—it is usually accurate.

On examination, your doctor will try to ascertain the location of the duct from which the discharge is emerging. A test called a galactogram may be ordered, in which a needle is inserted into the duct to pinpoint the source of the discharge. In the past, I considered the galactogram somewhat barbaric— but with newer, tiny catheters, it is less invasive.

Remember that the results of these tests are often inconclusive, and should not deter surgical excision of the duct or ducts. In preparation for this, one trick I've been using for some time involves a product called collodion—a sealant that is normally used to close scars after some forms of pediatric surgery. When you use this sealant once a day for about five days to occlude the nipple, the discharge is trapped and builds up inside the duct(s), at which point it becomes easy for your doctor to locate.

A surgical procedure can cause both cosmetic and sensation problems in the nipple and rarely impedes future breast-feeding.

Certainly any unusual discharge (*unusual for you*, that is) should be brought to your doctor's attention. Sometimes, discharge is associated with benign breast conditions, most commonly papillomatosis or duct ectasia (more on these later). As a rule, the older you are with papilloma, or nipple discharge, the greater the chance that it is associated with cancer. However, even in older women, nipple discharge is usually benign.

◆ ◆

◆ I HAVE A GREAT DEAL OF BREAST PAIN BEFORE I GET MY PERIOD. WHAT'S THE CAUSE?

There are many causes of mastalgia or breast pain, but about two-thirds of the time, it's related to the menstrual cycle—and termed "cyclical pain." The fluctuation in hormones that takes place throughout the menstrual cycle can cause varying

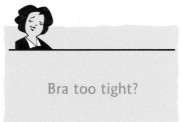

Bra too tight?

amounts of pain and sensitivity. The pain is usually related to the consistency of the breast at different points in the cycle—for instance, the increased nodularity and volume of the breast in the days just before your period begins can be associated with extreme tenderness. There are many theories as to why the breast is more tender at various points in the cycle—each relating to the relative amount of the hormones estrogen and progesterone that are present at that time. Usually the pain is in both breasts, and is poorly located—that is, it hurts all over the place. The pain often increases in severity from midcycle onward. Some women find that their breasts are so engorged and sensitive before menstruation that they can hardly be touched, and even putting on a bra is quite bothersome. Usually, the swelling and tenderness recede quickly within a day or so after menstruation starts.

◆ WHAT CAUSES BREAST PAIN OTHER THAN MENSTRUAL OR HORMONAL CHANGES?

One-third of breast pain is "noncyclical"—that is, it has nothing to do with the menstrual or hormonal cycles in your body.

Breast pain should be evaluated initially to exclude benign lesions of the breast, such as cysts, fibroadenomas, and other such problems that require aspiration or surgery. The broad term for many unrelated types of benign, noncyclical breast pain is MDAIDS—for mammary duct associated inflammatory disease sequence. Duct ectasia is one common benign problem that falls under this umbrella. It involves inflammation of the breast ducts, which can lead to scarring, which can in turn cause bad, localized breast pain. Another name for this problem is plasma cell mastitis (and others use the term periductal mastitis as well). A terrible cycle can develop in which the ducts fill with fluid, which leads to inflammation around the ducts, which in turn leads to scarring, all causing pain and further fluid buildup. Sometimes, it looks like an infection, and antibiotics are given; other times, it mimics cancer, and a biopsy is done.

MDAIDS can be chronic, lasting a few years and causing supersensitivity in the breasts. It's comforting that it's benign— but it sure isn't fun to live with. It tends to worsen in cold weather; the pain comes on abruptly and usually in the same site in the breast. Some women report a burning sensation behind the nipple. Often there is an associated sticky, green nipple discharge (which may contain bacteria). Sometimes, the nipples invert, or there is an accompanying mass in the areolar area around the nipple. In other cases there is an abscess (pus) or a fistula (a connection between the outside breast skin and an infection inside the breast). Some believe that there is an association between MDAIDS and cigarette smoking, especially in younger women—but this is controversial. (My personal take on that subject is that no one should smoke anyway, so it can't hurt to quit and find out if your breast pain abates!)

◆ How is **MDAIDS** treated?

For starters, reassurance is critical—women with this problem are often frightened and miserable, and finding out that the condition is benign and will likely recede with time can help a great deal. If there is an associated infection, antibiotics are needed. If there is an associated mass, surgery may be required. As for symptomatic relief, the following will help re-

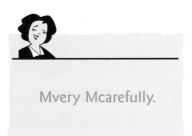

Mvery Mcarefully.

lieve pain: (1) mild analgesics and nonsteroidal anti-inflammatory drugs; (2) firm, supportive bras; (3) warm showers; and
(4) possibly smoking cessation.

◆ ARE THERE OTHER CAUSES OF NONCYCLICAL BREAST PAIN THAT ARE NOT RELATED TO MDAIDS?

Yes. For example, a less common type of noncyclical breast
pain is Tietze's syndrome, which involves an inflammation of
the cartilage where the rib cage meets the breastbone. With this
condition, you might experience pain *between* the breasts.
Usually nonsteroidal anti-inflammatory drugs will relieve the
pain and the problem will disappear with time.
    Less than 1 percent of the time, breast pain is caused by
trauma or by postbiopsy complications.

◆ MY DOCTOR SAYS I HAVE FIBROCYSTIC BREAST DISEASE. WHAT DOES THIS MEAN?

You'd be amazed how many
women are told that they have fibrocystic breast disease without any
firm documentation of the fact. It's
one of the most common "throw-
away" diagnoses about the breast.
Most women with working hor-

Call Dionne Warwick,
then open The
Fibrocystic Hotline.

mones have lumpy, bumpy, nodular breasts—and usually, this
is normal. But it is *not* fibrocystic breast *disease!* In fact, the
only accurate way to diagnose fibrocystic breasts—that is, the
whole host of breast changes in the chart on page 89—is with
a needle (or surgical) biopsy, or a sonogram test to reveal the
cysts. While some forms of fibrocystic breast disease *do* raise
the risk of breast cancer, common cysts *do not.* Too many doctors feel lumpy, granular, or nodular breasts and call them
"fibrocystic" based only on their physical examination. Insurance may call this a "pre-existing condition" and can refuse to
pay—and women understandably panic. But often, the diag-

nosis of fibrocystic breast disease is a fallacy. Always ask for the specific name of your condition, so that you can determine if it is in fact something to worry about.

"Fibrocystic breasts" encompasses many things, including cysts, fibroadenomas, radial scars, hyperplasia, duct ectasia, and other benign problems in the breast. Sonograms can diagnose cysts; sometimes mammograms can suggest—but not prove—that there is fibrocystic disease by demonstrating milk of calcium, when calcium is floating in cyst fluid, or diffusely scattered calcifications, which are commonly seen in a condition called sclerosing adenosis, also a form of fibrocystic disease. The bottom line: Fibrocystic breast *disease* cannot be diagnosed by your doctor's hands or imagination.

◆ SO WHAT ARE BREAST CYSTS?

Cysts are fluid-filled, which distinguishes them from other solid masses. They are extremely common in young, menstruating women, and in postmenopausal women taking hormone replacement therapy. In fact, about a third of women who have one cyst turn out to have additional cysts elsewhere in the breast—and half of the time you'll find cysts in the opposite breast as well. When I aspirate fluid from a cyst, it may appear yellow, bluish-black, or murky green, which I liken to muddy river water. As long as the cyst is not bloody, collapses completely, and has not recurred on reexamination of the breast, there's nothing to worry about. On the flip side of that coin, if the mass does not collapse or if there is blood present in it, I will recommend further testing.

Simple cysts do not require aspiration—if we're sure that's what they are. Sometimes, we do have to aspirate cysts—for instance, I will aspirate a lump I feel in the office, or if on a sonogram the cyst appears to be a combination of fluid and solid material (called a "complex" cyst), I will request a biopsy under

Breasts that are related.

the guidance of the sonogram machine. If a cyst is extremely large and interferes with my physical exam, I will aspirate it.

Sometimes, cysts do cause pain. For instance, when they abut on neighboring tissue, they can cause pressure and pain. Also, cysts can rupture, creating inflammation, which in turn can cause pain. So sometimes, I'll aspirate them to make women comfortable. But keep in mind, they can recur.

◆ CAN BREAST PAIN INDICATE CANCER?

Yes. I am troubled by the widespread myth that "if there's pain, there can't be cancer." It's always important to notify your doctor of any breast pain you may be having, so that he or she can do a complete workup and rule out the more common benign problems, as well as a potential cancer. Up to 15–20 percent of breast cancers may be associated with some degree of pain or discomfort.

Cyclical pain is less likely related to a serious problem than is constant pain. But there's no way to know just by guessing. Your doctor may recommend a mammogram (breast X ray) and will likely do a thorough physical examination of your breasts and take a detailed history of your discomfort to determine the underlying cause. Most cases of breast pain are *not* cancer. But that's no excuse to avoid a workup.

◆ MY FAMILY AND EVEN MY DOCTOR THINK I'M NEUROTIC AND IMAGINING MY BREAST PAIN. THIS IS VERY FRUSTRATING. CAN IT BE TRUE?

It's not only likely *un*true—it's terribly insulting and degrading to you and to women in general. You'd be surprised how common your complaint is. Usually, the accusation that women are imagining their breast pain is totally unfounded. Breast pain takes a terrible toll on your quality of life, making sex painful or impossible and seriously impairing your overall mood and ability to enjoy life. If you feel such pain, find a doctor who is willing to explore the many possible pathophysiologic causes—and one who respects you and takes your discomfort seriously. After a "pathologic" process is ruled out, and reassurance is given, 60–80 percent of women with breast pain require no further intervention.

◆ I READ IN A WOMEN'S MAGAZINE THAT I SHOULD AVOID CAFFEINE IN ORDER TO AVOID BREAST PAIN AND LUMPS. IS THIS TRUE?

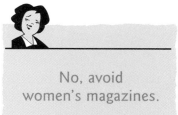

No, avoid women's magazines.

The *scientific* answer is "no"—studies have not substantiated a real connection between caffeine (methylxanthine) intake and breast pain or lumps. The *anecdotal* answer, however, is "yes"—there are lots of women out there who insist that caffeine promotes both breast discomfort and lumpiness. My advice is to see what works *for you*. If you have lumpy, painful breasts and you can live without your coffee, tea, caffeinated soda, or chocolate, for example, try giving them up. I know many women who find that their breasts feel better afterward, and I know many others who say the change made no difference whatsoever. Remember, there's always the placebo effect—that is, if your body *thinks* you have made a change for the better, you may in turn feel better. And there's nothing wrong with that! However, I confess that I enjoy the occasional cup (or more) of coffee, and haven't let breast sensations get in the way of it.

◆ I DO LOTS OF AEROBIC EXERCISE AND MY BREASTS BECOME VERY IRRITATED AFTERWARD. WHAT CAN I DO ABOUT THIS?

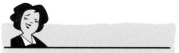

Sing softly to them in a calming voice.

Over-the-counter anti-inflammatory drugs, mild analgesics, warm showers, and well-fitting, supportive sports bras all can reduce discomfort. But certainly if you're relying even on mild pain medication more than once in a while, you should talk to your doctor about it. If you're doing high-impact aerobic exercise, you might consider switching to a lower-impact sport (e.g., walking or swimming instead of jogging, a stair-climbing machine instead of a treadmill, and so on). Your breasts will likely feel better as a result, and the joints throughout your body will also be grateful in the long run!

◆ WHAT CAN I DO TO RELIEVE MY BREAST PAIN?

That depends on the cause of your pain. So remember—if you're going to do something to relieve breast pain, don't do everything at once: try different remedies in isolation, so if you feel better, you'll know what works for you. There are a few general tips, however, that should help relieve your discomfort regardless of the cause:

• Use a well-fitting bra with good support. You'd be surprised how often you need to change bras—with weight gain or loss, changes in your breasts due to pregnancy or breast-feeding, or age-related changes. Avoid stretch strap bras; instead choose a bra with good, strong, adjustable straps. Some women sleep with a supportive sports bra for added support during the night—either on a regular basis, or premenstrually when their breasts are most tender.

• Ask your doctor if Motrin or other nonsteroidal anti-inflammatory drugs would be right for you. These drugs can help with many different types of breast pain—including premenstrual breast discomfort, inflammation in the breast or breast region due to Tietze's syndrome, or other musculoskeletal pain.

• Try abstaining from caffeine—but don't be surprised if you find that your breast pain persists. Caffeine, as discussed earlier, is a questionable cause of breast pain. Abstinence helps some women, but not others.

• Warm showers can help relieve breast pain from just about all causes. They are a valuable addition to any pain-relieving regimen.

• If your breast pain is primarily due to premenstrual fluid retention, you may gain some relief by avoiding salty foods for several days before you begin menstruating. Excessive dietary salt, which is common in the American woman's diet, tends to promote fluid retention throughout the body. Prepared, prepackaged, frozen, and "fast foods" tend to be the worst culprits; Chinese food, pizza, salty cheeses, processed lunch meats, canned goods, pickled items, and many kinds of chips and crackers are also loaded with salt. Avoid salt in your cooking and at the table. When possible, choose fresh fruits and vegetables; meats, poultry, and fish grilled with herbs but not with salt; simple oil and vinegar instead of salty dressings; and so on. Also be sure to drink a lot—at least eight 8-ounce glasses of water a day is a great tool for flushing excess fluid out of your body. Finally, exercise is another great tool for kicking excess fluid out of the body. While diuretic medications help reduce fluid retention, they can promote problems of their own, so don't start taking them without talking to your doctor about the right amount—*if any*—for you. Better to go the natural route.

• If your breast pain is cyclical (i.e., tied to your menstrual cycle), ask your doctor if about 3 grams of evening primrose oil, an herbal preparation, might help you. There is a theory that some breast pain is caused by a lack of essential fatty acids in the diet, so adding evening primrose oil—the richest known source of essential fatty acids—might relieve the pain. About a quarter of the women who try this preparation do find some relief. Some women complain of nausea and bloating while taking evening primrose oil, however.

• Some practitioners recommend the antigonadotropin hormone danazol to relieve breast pain. I do not advise it. Danazol may cause menstrual abnormalities in one of four women taking it, along with weight gain, nausea, and headaches. Another drug I don't recommend for the treatment of breast pain is bromocriptine, which can cause nausea, headaches, low blood pressure, or depression in one of three women.

If you are on hormone replacement therapy, ask your doctor about changing the combination of your prescription—this may help relieve breast pain.

In many cases of breast pain, the tincture of time is also good medicine. As a rule, breast pain peaks in women in their thirties and forties, and recedes thereafter. After menopause, for example, a great deal of breast pain disappears. So there may be a bright light at the end of the tunnel, even for women whose breast pain doesn't fully respond to treatment.

◆ I HAVE A SORE ON MY NIPPLE. CAN IT BE CANCER?

Yes, it could be cancer—but it doesn't have to be. Cancer of the nipple is known as Paget's disease—which is often associated with DCIS (ductal carcinoma-in-situ—more on DCIS on page 172). Paget's disease is another form of breast cancer that happens to appear on the nipple—not the areola around the nipple, but on the nipple itself. If your sore is on the areola only, it's not likely to be Paget's disease. Sometimes, however, it can spread, untreated, to the adjacent skin surrounding the nipple. Paget's disease can appear suddenly or gradually. Some women have associated cracking, ulceration, oozing, scaling, or crusting of the nipple as well.

Don't worry, it's probably just leprosy.

Years ago, more than half of women with Paget's disease presented with a nipple lesion and associated mass, but these days, thanks to earlier detection, Paget's disease is usually found when it is limited to the breast ducts.

Of course, there are *noncancerous*, common, scaly disorders of the skin of the breast as well—including eczema, psoriasis, herpes, jogger's nipple (from rubbing on the bra or shirt), and dermatitis. Dermatitis, or skin irritation and inflammation, can be triggered by allergy to nickel alloy in bra straps and hooks; latex; laundry detergent; or perfumes, for example. But always be sure to tell your doctor of *any* unusual lesions or bumps on your nipple—or elsewhere on your breast, for that matter—without delay. Do not apply topical creams or ointments without consulting your doctor, as these may mask Paget's disease.

◆ WHAT ARE THE TROUBLE SIGNS TO WATCH FOR IN MY OWN BREASTS?

You don't have to be a doctor to be a good guard dog for your own body. In fact, no one is better equipped than you to evaluate your body's changes, as you live inside it year in and year out. The more you know about your overall anatomy

They smoke, they chew tobacco, they stay out late, and they talk back.

and the anatomy of your breasts, the greater your chance of catching a problem early—and of alerting your doctor to that problem. So consider yourself your doctor's best ally.

Here are some key trouble signs to watch for in your breasts. They certainly do not guarantee that there is a cancer or other serious problem, but they should catch your attention so you, in turn, can bring them to the immediate attention of your doctor:

1. RECENT ASYMMETRY OF YOUR BREASTS: Many women have asymmetrical (different-sized) breasts, and this is perfectly normal. And there are other normal causes of breast asymmetry, including having surgery on one breast and not the other, or long-term breast-feeding on one side and not the other. But when your breasts are normally close in size, and then become asymmetrical without some obvious explanation, this can be a trouble sign. Be sure to discuss any such change with your doctor, as a breast can become smaller if a cancer is pulling the skin in and shortening the ducts. This can also create puckering on the skin of the breast.

2. PUCKERING, INDENTATION, OR RETRACTION OF THE SKIN: Puckering of the breast can indicate the existence of a cancer—perhaps one growing in or involving the connective tissue surrounding the breast ducts. Cancers close to the surface of the skin can cause puckering as well.

3. DIMPLING OF BREAST SKIN: This condition, known as peau d'orange or orange peel, may indicate the presence of a tumor that is blocking the lymph system and causing fluid accumulation under the skin. Be sure to bring it to your doctor's attention.

4. REDNESS OF THE BREAST SKIN: Redness does *not* necessarily indicate cancer—for instance, a woman who is breast-feeding and has redness, swelling, or warmth in a breast may have an infection or abscess. But if antibiotics fail to clear the problem, it's important to have your doctor confirm that no cancer or other underlying problem is present. A relatively rare form of breast cancer is called inflammatory breast cancer, and does involve redness and heat in the breast. When dimpling and redness appear together, this is more worrisome. Again, don't diagnose yourself—see your doctor.

5. ULCERATION OR ERODED SKIN ON THE BREAST: This is something I don't like to see on the surface of the breast, as it can indicate a cancer which is eroding the breast skin. Tell your doctor as soon as this sign appears.

6. RETRACTION OF THE NIPPLE: This must be differentiated from long-standing inverted nipples, which can be perfectly normal (see page 28). But a sudden, pronounced retraction of the nipple can indicate a cancer pulling the nipple inward. So show it to your doctor.

Other problems to look for are discussed earlier in this chapter, such as certain kinds of nipple discharge (page 34), and a sore on the nipple (page 44).

In the next chapter we will discuss how to screen your breasts for cancer and other common problems. Read it carefully for information on three key breast screening tools: your doctor's physical examination of your breasts; the breast self-exam, a monthly examination of your breasts which you do yourself and which will help you to find suspicious lumps or other irregularities in your breasts; and the lifesaving annual mammogram or breast X ray.

Had enough medical stuff for a while? Me too. Let's break for a pair of mammogram songs:

To the tune of "One Boy" from *Bye Bye Birdie*

Two breasts—
Two special breasts—
Two breasts so gorgeous—
They can't be ignored, just—
Two breasts—
Need a mammogram-am-am—

Two jugs—
Two pretty jugs—
You must protect 'em—
So early detect 'em—
Two jugs—
Should get checked, yes siree—

Now's time to find out—
How they're doin', don't live in doubt—
You'll be—
More healthy—
If you let your doctor see—

Two boobs—
Two splendid boobs—
Two boobs to X-ray—
Take care of your pecs, hey—
Two boobs—
Not one or three—
That's the way it should be—
And the T-shirt is free!

Sung by Christina Applegate and Rosie
to the tune of "Love and Marriage"

ROSIE: Check your boobies, check your boobies—
They're more precious than a million rubies—

CHRISTINA: The idea's a bright one—
So check the left and then the right one—

ROSIE: Test your mammaries, Test your mammaries—
Do it for your friends and for your families—

CHRISTINA: Look down—they're so perky—
To not protect 'em would be jerky!—

ROSIE: Squish squish squish and then you're finished—
It's just an X ray—

CHRISTINA: Squoosh, squoosh, squoosh, it can be more fun than—
A little foreplay—

ROSIE: Screen your ta-tas, screen your ta-tas—
If you're over forty you've just gotta—

CHRISTINA: It is not a bother—
Just check yourself—
For breast health—

BOTH: Then nag your sister and your mother!

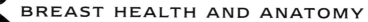

BREAST HEALTH AND ANATOMY

Y	S	F	F	Q	V	P	P	S	V	J	T	H	P
R	W	D	I	S	C	H	A	R	G	E	A	S	J
K	O	O	G	S	X	L	E	I	H	X	F	J	C
S	R	Q	R	G	V	E	O	W	W	D	S	H	N
D	U	C	T	S	V	P	N	U	R	S	I	N	G
J	Q	H	O	M	Q	R	L	T	S	T	D	Q	U
S	E	L	F	E	X	A	M	K	S	W	F	G	Y
N	I	P	P	L	E	W	T	A	L	D	F	Z	K
R	I	B	J	U	W	B	E	C	O	X	P	N	L
A	R	E	O	L	A	R	L	T	B	E	H	M	R
N	X	T	S	J	B	W	U	W	U	X	U	J	M
R	T	C	T	D	S	M	M	Y	L	W	Z	T	U
M	A	R	M	I	Z	Z	P	S	E	O	W	B	O
I	N	L	Z	H	G	E	J	Y	S	O	K	Q	R

Find and circle the following words:

AREOLA	DUCTS	LUMP	NURSING
BREAST	LOBULES	NIPPLE	SELF-EXAM
DISCHARGE			

2

THE BIG SQUEEZE:
Breast Screening

JULIA CHILD

I found the lump myself. I thought that something was wrong. It was about the size of a lima bean—I could feel it very definitely. It was around 1965, and the subject wasn't talked about. Not many people knew much about it. I went to my doctor and said, "I don't want to fool around; if it's malignant, please do what you think necessary." I didn't want to die. I was having a good time in my cooking career and I didn't want to have anything interfere with my pleasure in life.

The doctor said to come right in and had to operate on it. It was a complete mastectomy—they didn't have the lumpectomy in those days. The whole thing was lopped off. I thought, "You're a one-breasted woman, but you're alive." I didn't like being one-breasted, but I very much liked being alive. I know an older woman who had a lump, but she refused to have the surgery, she said she couldn't do that to her husband. She died two years later. My husband said, "I didn't marry you for your breast."

I do self-examination monthly and have a mammogram every year. I never even think about the cancer now, that was a long time ago. I have had no problems since. You're just stupid if you don't go to the doctor. It's up to you to take care of yourself, not up to anyone else. If you're not sure what you're feeling, go to the doctor anyway. Your life is in your own hands. I'm having too much fun not to care for myself.

◆ WHAT ARE THE GOALS OF BREAST SCREENING?

The major goal of breast cancer screening is to reduce the chance of

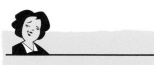

The two big nets at each end of the field.

dying from breast cancer by catching cancers as early as possible, when they are most treatable. Early detection also reduces the degree of disfigurement and other extensive procedures needed to treat breast cancer (again, because catching a cancer early means less extensive means can be used to treat it).

Screening does *not* reduce your chance of getting breast cancer (nor does it *increase* your risk, as popular myth may suggest). Screening increases the chance of catching an existing cancer as early as possible. Period. The tests are not perfect; the people who perform them are not perfect. But they are superb, lifesaving tools.

The three key tools for breast cancer screening are:
1. mammography—breast X rays;
2. physical examination of your breasts by your doctor; and
3. the breast self-exam—often called BSE.

◆ WHICH BREAST SCREENING TESTS SHOULD BE DONE, HOW OFTEN, AND WHEN?

Here is a list of which tests to have, and at what intervals. Keep in mind that if you are at increased risk of breast cancer because of certain factors such as your family history of the disease, or a pre-existing breast abnormality, your screening schedule may differ. Be sure to discuss this possibility with your doctor.

MAMMOGRAPHY:
WHO?—ALL WOMEN FORTY AND OVER
HOW OFTEN?—EVERY YEAR
WHEN?—IF YOU MENSTRUATE, 7–10 DAYS AFTER YOU BEGIN YOUR MENSTRUAL PERIOD; OTHERWISE, NEAR YOUR BIRTHDAY IS A GOOD REMINDER AND A GREAT PRESENT TO YOURSELF

In women with a first-degree relative with premenopausal breast cancer, screening should begin ten years earlier than the age at which cancer was diagnosed in that relative, but not earlier than twenty-five years of age.

PHYSICAL EXAMINATION OF YOUR BREASTS BY A DOCTOR:

WHO?—ALL WOMEN

HOW OFTEN?—EVERY YEAR

WHEN?—IF YOU MENSTRUATE, 7–10 DAYS AFTER YOUR PERIOD BEGINS, WHEN YOUR BREASTS ARE MOST COMFORTABLE; OTHERWISE, ANYTIME

BREAST SELF-EXAM (BSE):

WHO?—ALL WOMEN TWENTY AND OVER

HOW OFTEN?—EVERY MONTH

WHEN?—SAME TIME EACH MONTH; IF YOU MENSTRUATE, 7–10 DAYS AFTER YOUR PERIOD BEGINS

TOP 5 REASONS TO HAVE A REGULAR BREAST EXAM BY YOUR DOCTOR:

1. Because the doctor's really cute.

2. Where else can you be guaranteed to get felt up?

3. It's fun and you don't have to speak to your doctor again for a whole year.

4. When else will your insurance cover entertainment?

5. It's fun to watch your doctor panic while, during your examination, you dreamily ask, "Do you love me?"

◆ WHY IS THE MAMMOGRAM IMPORTANT?

The mammogram, which is an X-ray examination of the breast, is the best tool we have for detecting breast cancers while they are still too tiny to be felt. This is known as the "pre-clinical phase." When you catch cancer early, your outlook for survival is greatest. There are tens of thousands of women alive today because mammograms caught their cancers before they spread.

The preclinical phase is different for women at different ages, and also varies for tumors with different patterns and varying degrees of aggressiveness. For instance, the *average* time between the appearance of a cancer on a mammogram and when it can be felt is 1.7 years for women aged forty to forty-nine; for women fifty to fifty-nine, it is longer—at between 3.3 and 3.8 years. In either case, you can see that there is an im-

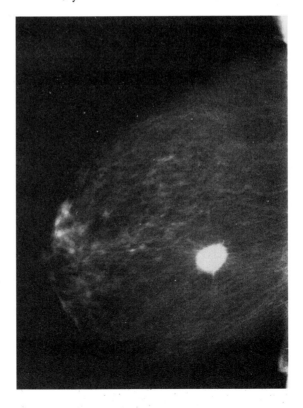

This is a cancer in a seventy-year-old woman.

◆ ◆

portant window during which the mammogram can do the detective work that neither you, nor your doctor, can do with your fingers.

◆ SHOULD I PREPARE FOR MY MAMMOGRAM IN ANY SPECIAL WAY?

Yes. The American Cancer Society recommends the following measures before your breast X ray. Some are for convenience only; others affect the quality of the test.

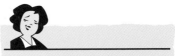

Marinate them in teriyaki sauce overnight.

• Wear a two-piece outfit so you will only have to remove your top.

• Do not use deodorant, talcum powder, or lotion under your arms or near the breasts that day. These products can show up on the X-ray picture and mimic or hide breast abnormalities.

• Bring the name, address, and phone number of your doctor or other health care provider. This way the doctors at your mammography center can communicate any important information to your regular physician—or ask important questions that might clarify a finding on your X ray. Also, write a list of questions you may forget to ask.

• Bring your previous mammography films, as well as the radiologist's report if it was not done at the same facility, and any past pathology reports. Your new mammogram can then be compared with your old one(s) to see if any meaningful changes have developed. Also bring a list of the places and dates of any previous mammograms, biopsies, or other breast treatments you have received. Your original films belong to the center where they were taken, but if you are moving to another city or no longer plan to use the facility, you should keep the films yourself (place them in cold storage).

Also note: If you are worried about discomfort during the mammogram, you might want to take a mild over-the-counter painkiller about an hour before the test. Rarely, I will give a stronger prescription medicine for anxiety, for women who are particularly frightened and will not have the test without it.

And remember: Don't settle for the "no news is good news" maxim when it comes to your mammogram results. Before you leave, ask the technician about when you should expect to receive the results of your test. It usually takes about ten days or less, but ideally women should be given their results before they leave the facility (this is unfortunately done quite rarely). If you haven't heard anything by then, pick up the phone and call for your results. A terrific new law requires mammography

LIMERICKS

You may think that you're sitting pretty
But here is the real nitty-gritty
You're in for a whammo
If you don't go mammo
Take care of your left and right titty!

There once was a woman named Millie
Who thought breast exams were quite silly
She stalled and she stalled
Till her best friend called
They both went, and then shared some chili.

A woman once got very jumpy
Because she detected a lump-y
She saw her M.D.
Who did tests 1-2-3
And now she is happy, not grumpy.

facilities to notify patients directly—in lay terms—of the results of their mammograms.

◆ DOES MAMMOGRAPHY HURT?

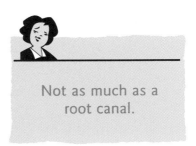

Not as much as a root canal.

Most women would describe the feeling as mild discomfort at the worst—while others aren't bothered at all. The machine compresses or flattens the breasts, so there is a sensation of pressure, but there should not be pain. This compression lasts for only a few seconds. The key is to have the test done at a time of the month when your breasts are the least sensitive. For instance, many women find that their breasts are highly sensitive shortly before menstruation—making this a bad time to have a mammogram done. A few days after your period is finished, however, is usually the *least* sensitive time for the breasts, and therefore a great time to schedule your mammogram. This isn't always possible, though, as many mammography facilities are quite heavily booked.

◆ I'VE HEARD THAT MAMMOGRAPHY RESULTS CAN BE WRONG. IS THIS TRUE?

Mammography is an excellent tool, but no test—including this one—is perfect. There are both "false negatives" (cases in which cancer is diagnosed within one year of a normal mammogram) and "false positives" (cases in which patients are called back for additional tests, and these tests indicate no cancer present). How common are these errors? About 1 in 4 invasive breast cancers is missed by mammography in women forty to forty-nine years of age. The test is more accurate for women aged fifty to fifty-nine: in this group, only about 1 out of 10 invasive breast cancers is missed by mammography. But the bright side of these statistics is that three-fourths of cancers in

TOP 5 THINGS TO DO AFTER GETTING A MAMMOGRAM:

1. Tuck your boobs into your pants and go the hell home!

2. Get your X rays made into wallet-size.

3. McDonald's.

4. Go out through the waiting room shouting, "I got a mammogram!" and demanding applause.

5. Cry until the technician gives you a lollipop.

younger women are caught, and 9 of 10 cancers in older women are caught with mammography. As for false positives—about 10 percent of all screening mammograms are read as abnormal, which creates the need for additional tests such as repeat mammograms, ultrasound, needle aspiration, core biopsy, or surgical biopsy. It is estimated that 1 in 4 women aged forty to sixty-nine who have an average of four mammograms over a ten-year period will require additional evaluation of some kind. That's a pretty big number. However, most women would trade the discomfort, cost, and inconvenience of extra testing for an accurate diagnosis.

◆ ISN'T THERE A RISK OF GETTING TOO MUCH RADIATION FROM A MAMMOGRAM?

Not anymore. In the old days, mammography machines gave off more radiation than they do today. The current machines give extremely low doses of radiation—much less, in fact, than many activities that women don't fear at all. For example, the amount of radiation exposure in a mammogram is about the same as what you get when flying across the U.S. and back in a commercial jet. And your dentist exposes you to more radiation during a routine series of X rays in your mouth. So there's no reason to worry.

◆ Why was there so much controversy over the use of mammography in younger women?

When you say "younger women," you're referring to women aged forty to forty-nine—since this is the group that was once controversial in terms of mammography screening. Let me stress that the question is no longer open: *All women starting at age forty should have mammograms every single year.*

There was a great hoopla a few years ago when several of the leading breast cancer policy-setting organizations disagreed over whether there was value in screening younger women with mammography. Several organizations said *not* to screen younger women, while the American Cancer Society (ACS) said to screen them every one to two years. But many leading scientists and clinicians harshly criticized the studies that suggested that mammography was not valuable in younger women. There were serious flaws in the research, including the type of mammography machines that were used and the basic study design. The National Cancer Institute and other groups withdrew their recommendation against mammography in younger women. And the ACS maintained, as it always has, that mammography is needed for younger women—and *upped* their recommendation to *every year for all women forty and over.*

The bottom line is that the benefits of screening outweigh the risks of mammography in this age group. What do I mean by "the risks"? Let me explain. The younger a woman is, the more dense her breasts usually are. This density can make breasts harder to "read" with a mammogram. As a result, there are more false positives in younger women—that is, doctors become worried about lots of images that appear on the mammogram, and send the women for further testing, sometimes invasive testing, which may prove to be unnecessary and can provoke great anxiety. These additional tests carry risks of their own. For example, younger women are sometimes given needle biopsies, or other invasive procedures, which often turn out to show that *no* cancer is present. However—and this is a big however—most women would say that in the long run, it's preferable to have an extra (albeit unpleasant) biopsy in order to rule out cancer than to leave the lesion untested and hope for the best.

Also, because breast cancer tends to be more aggressive in younger women (this is not always the case, but often is so), mammography can be even more critical in this group of women. The sooner an aggressive cancer is found, the sooner tough cancer-fighting therapies can be started. Lost time in treatment of a young woman's cancer can be even more costly than in an older woman. So it's absolutely vital to have your mammogram every year starting at age forty. Finally, if you follow the guidelines for smart mammography screening listed in the answer that follows, you'll help your doctors to avoid making mistakes in reading your X-ray films. For example, by bringing along your mammograms from recent years so that your doctor can compare your new and older films, you will help eliminate the possibility that the same old benign lesion will be retested.

How should I go about choosing a good mammography center?

Select a facility that is certified by the FDA (U.S. Food and Drug Administration) and that is accredited by the ACR (American College of Radiologists) or by the states of Arkansas, California, or Iowa. Ask to see a copy of these certificates. Thanks to a new law enacted in 1994, called the Mammography Quality Standards Act, it is against the law to perform mammography in the U.S. without an FDA certificate. This helps insure that the facility meets certain basic standards for both safety and quality.

Accreditation covers all aspects of the mammography process, including:

- the mammography machines
- the personnel who perform the test (radiologic mammography technologists)
- those who read and interpret the test results (radiologists, also called mammographers), and
- those who manage the mammography equipment itself (medical physicists).

The more mammograms the center does, the better—ideally, choose one that specializes in mammography, or at least does a large number of mammograms each day. See page 267 in the Resources section for details on how to find an FDA-certified mammography center near you.

The recall rate—that is, the rate of calling women back for extra tests—should be no more than 1 in 10 women. Ideally, the facility will do what's known as a "wet read," in which they take a look at the mammography films and determine on the spot whether women will need additional X-ray views. And in cases where women are known to have particular abnormalities in the breast, special kinds of views should be taken. For instance, with microcalcifications, special magnification films *may* need to be done to take a closer look at them. Sometimes, a mass on a mammogram may need to be compressed, because it could represent superimposed breast tissue. This is yet another situation in which communication is so critical between your various health care providers. If your regular physician or health care provider communicates special needs to the personnel at the mammography center, your mammogram and its subsequent interpretation will be best customized to your case. And that can mean the difference between catching an early cancer and missing it.

◆ When and why are sonograms used for breast screening?

There are places that uses sonograms for breast screening, but this is very controversial. I personally recommend sonography for *diagnostic* purposes—not for initial screening. For instance, sonograms are useful to study a mass that I feel in a pregnant or breast-feeding woman, and they are helpful in determining if a mass located on a mammogram is solid or cystic. I also find sonograms useful in guiding some interventional procedures, or sometimes for taking a look at breast implants (though MRI is better for looking at implant rupture).

◆ My last mammogram was normal. Why should I bother having one year after year?

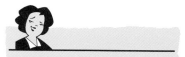

I brushed my teeth yesterday, why should I bother brushing day after day?

Breast cancer can appear at any time. This is why you must have a new mammogram every year. Be thankful that you have older, normal breast X rays that your doctors can use for means of comparison with your new films. This makes it easier to detect new changes in the breast that could indicate the development of a cancer or some other problem. Also, don't forget that if you *feel* a lump—even if your mammogram was normal—you should still ask your doctor for a further workup. About 10 percent of breast cancers are detected only by physical examination.

◆ I'm over sixty-five, why should I bother with mammograms?

Actually, the risk of breast cancer increases with age. Age is one of the biggest risk factors for breast cancer, so a woman is never in the clear. It's absolutely critical that you have a mammogram every year. If you catch a cancer early, it will be easier to treat, and you will have more treatment options, including the chance to save your breast. There is anecdotal evidence that doctors often fail to refer older women to get mammograms. Even if your doctor doesn't press you to do so, it can be lifesaving.

MAMMOGRAMS ARE COSTLY. HOW AM I SUPPOSED TO PAY FOR ONE EVERY YEAR?

The average mammogram costs about $100–$250. Most insurance companies, plus Medicaid and Medicare, pay for all or part of the procedure every year. But keep this in mind: there are many programs out there to help women with limited financial means to get regular mammograms at reduced cost, or even for free. For example, October has been designated "Breast Cancer Awareness Month," and during this month there are free or low-cost mammography screening programs all over the country. Your own local hospital or clinic may take part in such a program—be sure to call and ask about it. The American Cancer Society also can help you to locate such a cost-saving program in your area.

I AM EXTREMELY FLAT-CHESTED. DOES THIS MAKE IT HARDER TO GET AN ACCURATE MAMMOGRAM?

Yes, it can be harder—but you can certainly still get a good image. The key is to have an experienced technologist who knows the best positioning to get a clear image. The same holds for women with a curvature of the spine, or a protruding or indented chest—proper positioning is critical to getting a good mammogram.

No ONE IN MY FAMILY HAS BREAST CANCER. WHY SHOULD I HAVE REGULAR MAMMOGRAMS?

It is unfortunately a prevalent myth that people with no family history of breast cancer don't have to worry about this disease. But the hard truth is that about 9 in 10 cases of breast cancer occur in women with *no* family history of the disease. True, having a first-degree relative with breast cancer—i.e., a mother, sister, or daughter—increases your risk of getting breast cancer yourself. But there are many other risk factors for breast cancer—some known, and some unknown. Mammography is a test for all women forty and over, regardless of their family history of breast cancer.

◆ HOW EXACTLY SHOULD I DO THE BREAST SELF-EXAM?

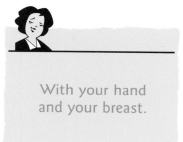

With your hand and your breast.

There are several techniques, including one in which you go round and round the breasts in a circular motion, and another in which you do a series of up-and-down strip searches of the breast, and pie-shaped wedges. I strongly prefer the up-and-down (vertical) strip search method, as it tends to cover all of the breast tissue. With the circular method, it's easier to miss a ring of breast tissue as you're going round and round.

The Mammacare company in Gainesville, Florida, sells a very useful breast model that contains several simulated breast tumors and other lumps. You can use the model to practice the breast self-exam and to get a better idea of what to feel inside the breast.

I sometimes give a small test breast model (with two masses inside) to women in my office. It can be purchased through Health Edco in Waco, Texas.

There are two key concepts involved in the proper use of this method of breast self-exam. The first one involves using three different levels of pressure when feeling the breasts. The idea is to check the breast at various depths, rather than doing one simple check in which you try to push all the way down inside the breast.

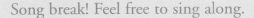

Song break! Feel free to sing along.

To the theme song of *I Love Lucy*

I love boobies
Now go check yours
They're two buddies
You can't ignore
I know you're scared and you dread it
But if you hold out, you might regret it

Boobies big and small all need care
Let your doc see what's under there
You've such a pretty set
And your best bet
Is that you get
A mammogram-am-am-am-am-am-am!

To the theme song of *The Addams Family*

Good health is what you wish 'em
Go squash 'em and then squish 'em
Don't be a jelly fish 'em
Go get a mammogram!

Da da da da squash squash
Da da da da squish squish

The whole thing, ma'am, is easy
No reason to be queasy
It's more fun than Parcheesi
Go get a mammogram!

Da da da da squash squash
Da da da da squish squish

It's all about detection
So make the doc connection
And save your prized collection
Go get a mammogram!

Da da da da squash squash
Da da da da squish squish

If you're a fuddy duddy
Then why not take a buddy
These aren't Silly Putty
Go get a mammogram!

Da da da da squash squash
Da da da da squish squish

If forty or more you be
Then better be a doo-bee
And take care of your boobies
Go get a mammogram!

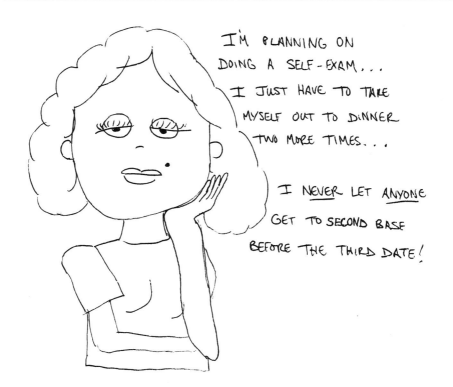

I'M PLANNING ON DOING A SELF-EXAM... I JUST HAVE TO TAKE MYSELF OUT TO DINNER TWO MORE TIMES...

I NEVER LET ANYONE GET TO SECOND BASE BEFORE THE THIRD DATE!

CAN YOU DESCRIBE HOW I SHOULD USE MY FINGERS TO EXAMINE MY BREASTS?

Using the pads of your fingers, first apply light pressure to the breast, as you are checking the area just slightly underneath the breast skin's surface. Next, apply medium pressure to the breast, checking about midway inside the breast. And finally, apply deep pressure, feeling for the area deepest in the breast. You should use these three pressures as you examine your breasts.

The second critical concept in doing the breast self-exam is to cover *all* of your breast tissue, and as I mentioned earlier in this chapter, that tissue can cover a lot more ground than most women realize. Breast tissue often extends up to the collarbone; down to the rib cage or even below the rib cage and bra line; and all the way to each underarm. Your self-exam should cover this landscape as well. And most important, do not allow your fingers to stop or lift away from your breast at any point in the middle of the exam. Here's what to do:

Lie on your side, but twist back a bit so your breast falls as flat as possible on your chest, rather than hanging down toward the floor. This helps you to cover more surface area and allows you to apply firm pressure against a hard surface. Now you can begin your "strip search" of the breast. Do your light, medium, and deep presses in straight lines moving in vertical lines from your collarbone down to below your bra line and covering the

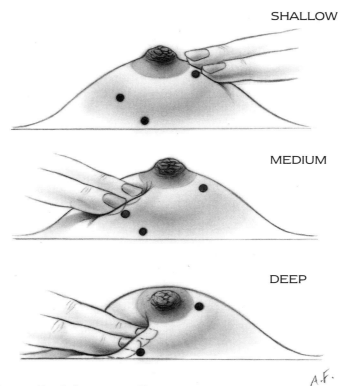

SHALLOW

MEDIUM

DEEP

A.F.

Three Pressure Levels for Breast Self-Exam

◆   ◆   ◆   ◆   ◆   ◆   ◆   ◆   ◆   ◆   ◆   ◆   ◆   ◆   ◆   ◆   ◆   ◆   ◆   ◆

area from the armpit to the breastbone. Use the left arm to check the right breast and vice versa. You might want to use lotion or powder to help you move over the breast smoothly.

Correct Positioning for Breast Self-Exam

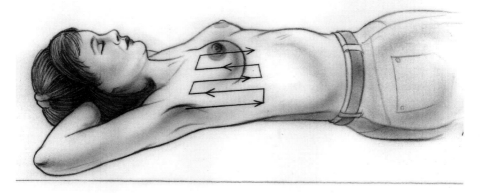

Strip Search Lines for Breast Self-Exam

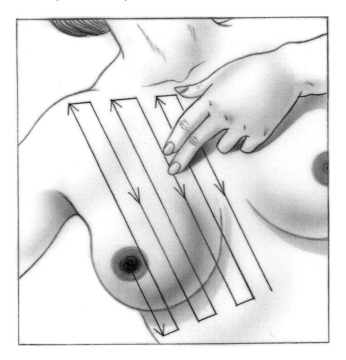

Examine breasts one at a time, and examine both breasts every time. And do the exam every month. With time, you will become intimately familiar with the architecture of your breasts, and well equipped to tell your doctor about any new changes in them. If you feel a new potential "abnormality," check the other breast in the same region to see if it's symmetrical.

◆ IS THERE A BETTER OR WORSE TIME TO DO THE BREAST SELF-EXAM EACH MONTH?

It's useful to do the breast self-exam at the same time each month, because the breasts tend to change (as a result of changing hormones) throughout a woman's monthly cycle. If you have a regular menstrual cycle, then the best time to do the breast self-exam is about seven to ten days after your period begins each month. At this time, your breasts are the least lumpy and the least tender to the touch.

If you *don't* have regular monthly periods, then try to do your breast self-exam on the same day each month—for example, on the first of every month, the day you pay your monthly bills, your bridge game, or something else you won't forget.

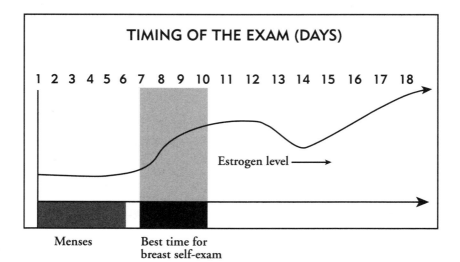

TIMING OF THE EXAM (DAYS)

1 2 3 4 5 6 7 8 9 10 11 12 13 14 15 16 17 18

Estrogen level ⟶

Menses

Best time for
breast self-exam

BREAST SELF-EXAMINATION SONG

To the tune of "Baby Face"

Booby test—
     You've got to do a little booby test—
     Though mates and nursing children touch your breast—
     I attest—
     You need self-inspection—
     For that ear-ly detection—

Booby test—
     When in the shower you must check those lovely pecs—
     Hey don't be scared or smug—
     Give yourself healthy jugs—
     Do a frequent booby test!

◆ CAN YOU GIVE ME SOME GENERAL GUIDELINES ON WHAT TO "FEEL" FOR IN MY BREASTS?

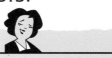

Most women's breasts have lots of bumpy or nodular areas in them. Only young girls' breasts are perfectly smooth. The goal in checking your breasts is to find dominant lumps—something that stands out and that is not symmetrical with the other breast. Symmetry is very important: if you find the same lump in the other breast, it's usually normal.

While doing it, think of the happy ending to "The Princess and the Pea."

Search for lumps that are hard, irregular in shape, not painful, and not mobile (i.e., something that's attached to the skin or muscle and that doesn't move). These can be (but aren't always) problem signs, and should be brought to your doctor's attention. The lump can be in the breast area, under the arm, or anywhere else in the region. Also, if such a lump is associated with a change on the skin of your breast, tell your doctor.

On the contrary, lumps that are mobile, smooth, painful, and unattached are generally nothing to worry about, but *always* need investigation. Certainly painful lumps *can* be cancerous. Always tell your doctor of a new lump.

Finally, remember that breast tumors appear in areas other than the breast itself. Breast tissue can extend all the way over to the underarm; up to the collarbone; and down to the rib cage.

The bottom line is, you can't be perfect. Even doctors trained in evaluating breast lumps are wrong up to 30 percent of the time when making judgments about what they feel in their patients' breasts. You can't expect much more of yourself. Do the best you can—and bring anything suspicious to your doctor's attention.

◆ WHY DO SOME DOCTORS FEEL THE BREAST SELF-EXAM IS NOT WORTHWHILE?

There is some controversy over the breast self-exam, as no rigorous long-term study has ever shown that the exam saves lives. But I happen to believe—and I am not alone—that the problem lies not with the test itself, but with the way women do it. Because so few people know how to do the breast self-exam properly (or they don't do it every month, or they don't do it at all), it's hard to really measure the effectiveness of the test *done right*. I have personally seen the wonderful results when a woman does the exam properly, catches a cancer early, and ends up with a terrific prognosis as a result. So unless doing the exam makes you feel too uncomfortable and anxious, I urge you to keep your faith in the test, learn how to do it right, and practice, practice, practice every month.

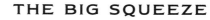

THE BIG SQUEEZE

V	A	T	M	O	U	S	S	P	U	G	S	F	V	R	T
I	S	L	A	R	S	T	Q	H	L	L	B	O	I	E	R
P	M	O	O	G	P	L	U	Y	R	R	O	R	L	Z	E
B	S	E	N	O	M	U	M	S	E	A	B	M	N	E	A
R	M	U	M	A	M	E	E	A	W	M	B	A	A	E	L
E	H	D	A	M	S	A	S	L	R	B	R	R	P	U	P
T	L	E	F	I	N	T	E	U	W	G	F	M	S	Q	R
V	W	U	V	F	I	L	Z	M	X	S	O	A	C	S	A
S	R	E	M	E	T	L	E	B	R	E	R	M	R	P	S
T	Y	T	E	P	A	K	B	S	A	V	T	T	M	O	T
R	H	I	N	M	O	N	T	H	L	Y	Y	S	A	A	O
A	G	E	L	A	V	X	R	M	P	E	O	S	R	R	M
W	S	Y	E	O	U	G	E	O	H	A	R	L	M	G	A
N	Q	U	E	E	N	L	A	N	Y	R	T	X	O	T	M
Q	R	A	P	H	Y	S	I	C	A	L	F	A	C	L	O
U	R	N	T	U	K	L	X	R	A	Y	R	X	R	A	C

Find and circle the following words:

BSE	PHYSICAL	MAMMOGRAM
MONTHLY	SQUEEZE	FORTY
X RAY	BREAST	
YEARLY	LUMP	

3

KNOWING YOUR RISK:
What Causes Breast Cancer?

DIAHANN CARROLL

I was absolutely shocked when I was diagnosed. I was so positive that I was not even in the running: I never thought that I was a candidate for cancer. There had been no breast cancer in my family that I was aware of, and I've been healthy and exercised all of my life. It was very surreal when my doctor said that word. He started to say that the good news was that it was very small, it's less than a centimeter, etc., etc., but I had to stop him then and there. I literally said to him, "Are you saying that I have cancer?" and he said, "Yes." He then started telling me about the type of cancer I had, and I said, "You have to allow me to hang up, because I don't . . . I can't even hear you now."

I walked around and around and around for maybe twenty minutes, a half-hour, and then I called my doctor back and said, "Start at the beginning. What is it I have to know? I'm going to center myself for a moment and I'm going to make some notes as you speak, so that it will become real for me." He then told me that I had cancer, that it was less than a square centimeter, and that he recommended seven weeks of radiation.

I had planned on taking notes as he was speaking, but I just could not write . . . I could not do anything.

Diahann Carroll's best advice:

One of the most important things I can say to women is doctors are just human beings. If you feel you can't get information from them, or if they aren't being helpful, tell them that you need more information than you've been given. Don't be intimidated by your doctors, by their degrees . . . remember, they are there to help you.

I've discovered that many women are afraid to ask their doctor questions, are afraid to say, "What do you mean by that?" or "I don't understand." That fear renders them speechless.

That's why I've become involved with Rite-Aid's Mother's Day Mammograms (a national program designed to make sure that all women have access to the preventive health benefits of regular mammograms. The program reaches out to women across the country who do not have the money and/or health insurance for a mammogram and connects them with local health care providers that offer the valuable screening test free of charge.) Women particularly find comfort in the program because they can dial the number (1-888-RITE-NOW) and have a discussion with someone who will give them the information they require and point them in the right direction.

I think this program will be particularly valuable to the many African American communities throughout the country, where, unfortunately, there is a lack of education about breast cancer. The proper education allows people to think and ask questions. Many black men are equally afraid when they hear about prostate cancer. This fact is probably due to the emotional "survival kit" one develops in the black community. Part of the survival kit is denial, the belief that "whatever it is, it will go away." Sadly, we've found that women in black and Hispanic communities, where the income is usually insufficient, believe that they can't afford to have cancer, therefore, they just deny the possibility of getting cancer.

◆ I CAN'T SEEM TO AVOID THAT TERRIBLE STATISTIC THAT 1 IN 8 WOMEN WILL GET BREAST CANCER. IS THIS REALLY TRUE?

Statistics are very useful in some cases, but very misleading and frightening in others. In this case, the widely publicized statistic that 1 in 8 women will get breast cancer is true, but not in the way most women think about risk. The fact is, 1 in 8 women will develop breast

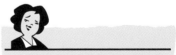

Yes. Four out of five dentists who recommend gum to their patients chew Trident.

cancer over the course of an eighty-five-year lifetime—not at any single point in time. So if you're forty-five, your chance of getting breast cancer this year is not 1 in 8 (which is exactly what most women believe). In fact, your chance of getting breast cancer at the age of forty-five is almost twelve times less—at 1 in 93. The table below comes from the National Cancer Institute, and gives a more realistic picture of the average risk of getting breast cancer at various ages. Remember, these are averages. But they're certainly more useful than the scary 1 in 8 number that has been implied to affect every woman at every age.

> **YOUR RISK OF GETTING BREAST CANCER AT VARIOUS AGES:**
>
> By age twenty-five: 1 in 19,608
> By age thirty: 1 in 2,525
> By age thirty-five: 1 in 622
> By age forty: 1 in 217
> By age forty-five: 1 in 93
> By age fifty: 1 in 50
> By age fifty-five: 1 in 33
> By age sixty: 1 in 24
> By age sixty-five: 1 in 17
> By age seventy: 1 in 14
> By age seventy-five: 1 in 11
> By age eighty: 1 in 10
> By age eighty-five: 1 in 8

If you live until the age of 120, your chance of getting breast cancer reaches that publicized 1 in 8 figure. Most women I know would readily gain an extra forty years of life expectancy in exchange for this risk.

I HAVE HEARD THAT GETTING YOUR PERIOD AT A YOUNG AGE, AND REACHING MENOPAUSE LATE, BOTH INCREASE THE RISK OF BREAST CANCER. IS THIS TRUE, AND WHY?

Yes, it's true—early menstruation (before age twelve) and late menopause (after age fifty-five) both increase the risk of breast cancer. If you get your period before age twelve, your risk is 30 percent greater than a woman who first menstruates after that age. And if

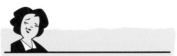

Ask your friends at the tampon company.

you reach menopause after age fifty-five, and have a total of more than forty menstruating years, your risk of breast cancer is doubled. The reason? It is believed that the longer your body is exposed to the hormone estrogen, the greater your risk of breast cancer. It's worth noting that the risk of breast cancer is greater for women who have regular, monthly menstrual periods than for those who have occasional or rare periods. A young woman who first menstruates at age eleven but who doesn't kick in to having regular monthly periods for several years may be at lower risk than one who gets her period at thirteen but immediately starts monthly periods. The difference is in the body's total exposure to estrogen—the more estrogen, the greater the risk. (That said, however, not *all* kinds of estrogen are bad—as we will discuss in several places throughout this book.)

Some ask why older women—who no longer produce much estrogen—have a higher risk of breast cancer than younger women have. The answer is quite simple: it's both the *duration* and *intensity* of estrogen exposure that appear to increase risk—exposure that accrues over a lifetime. Also, as we will discuss in this chapter, there are other, nonestrogen risk factors for breast cancer that come into play as well.

◆ IF I FALL INTO A HIGH-RISK CATEGORY, WHAT SHOULD I DO?

The important thing to keep in mind is that we're talking about what scientists call "relative risk"—not "absolute risk"—which means that you are relatively more likely to get breast cancer than women who don't have a given risk factor, but by no means are you guaranteed to get

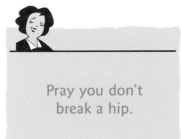

Pray you don't break a hip.

it! Most women who get breast cancer have *no* identifiable risk factor for the disease. So if you're reading this and find that you fit any particular risk factor category in this chapter, certainly don't panic. It just may be valuable for you, and your doctor, to be aware of any additional risk you have as a result of things beyond your control—or because of lifestyle factors.

Interestingly, there are ways to modify some estrogen-related risk factors. For example, women who exercise vigorously early in life—say, in school sports—tend to menstruate later than those who are more sedentary. Or, for another example, if you have a number of full-term pregnancies and breast-feed afterward, you will reduce the number of menstrual cycles you experience throughout your lifetime, thereby reducing your risk. We'll look more closely at the impact of exercise, diet, pregnancy, breast-feeding, and other lifestyle factors later in this chapter. But it is interesting to see how these processes all tie together to increase, or reduce, the risk of breast cancer over a woman's lifetime.

MY MOTHER'S FRIEND SAYS HER BREAST CANCER WAS CAUSED BY RADIATION TREATMENTS FOR A BIRTHMARK ON HER CHEST DURING CHILDHOOD. HOW MUCH AND WHAT KIND OF RADIATION IS RISKY?

In the past, many people were treated with repeated exposures to *ionizing* radiation for a variety of problems including acne and other skin lesions, an enlarged thymus, tuberculosis, breast infections, and other reasons. The sad legacy of these exposures, for many women, has been breast cancer (and other cancers as well)—even decades later. The most extreme cases, of course, can be seen when you look at the victims of disasters such as the atomic explosions in Japan, the Chernobyl nuclear accident, and other radiation crises. Cancers of many kinds, including breast and thyroid cancer, are more common among those exposed to these high doses of radiation.

I always recommend that women who had some type of radiation therapy—e.g., for Hodgkin's disease—start careful screening for breast cancer no more than eight years after completion of treatment (but not before age twenty-five). Certainly most of these women will *not* develop breast cancer, but it's wise to be especially vigilant so that in the event a breast cancer does develop, it will likely be caught early, when it is most easily treatable.

There is some evidence that the developing breast is more susceptible to permanent damage from radiation exposure than is the mature breast. For instance, during a female baby's development in the womb and later during puberty (two periods during which the breasts are under fast development or growth and change), the risk of radiation exposure and its impact on the risk of breast cancer may be greatest. So while it is always important to avoid radiation exposure, it is especially critical at certain times of life.

◆ MY MOTHER TOOK THE DRUG DES IN THE 1950S. IS SHE—AND AM I—MORE LIKELY TO GET BREAST CANCER AS A RESULT?

Yes. Even though your mother probably took DES for only a few months during pregnancy, you are both at somewhat greater risk of developing breast cancer as a result. DES (diethylstilbestrol) was an estrogenic drug taken by many women in the 1940s through the 1960s in the mistaken belief that it would cut their risk of miscarriage. It is thought that because DES exposure occurred during a time of rapid breast change and growth (during pregnancy for the mother, and during prenatal development for the baby), the impact on breast cancer risk may be greater than it would be at other times. After all, estrogen is present in great amounts during pregnancy without the addition of DES. But adding another estrogen source to the body, whether from drugs or the environment, might be the straw that breaks the camel's back for some women.

For the pregnant woman who took DES herself, the risk of breast cancer is 50 percent greater than for women who did not take the drug. For the baby exposed in utero, the risk is less well established, since these women are only now coming of breast cancer age. But early studies suggest that the risk of breast cancer is increased, as is the risk of a rare vaginal cancer in young women called clear cell adenocarcinoma. Screening of the breast and cervix is essential for these women.

◆ I NEVER HAD BIOLOGICAL CHILDREN. DOES THIS PUT ME AT GREATER RISK OF BREAST CANCER?

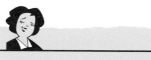

Here's a case in which the impact of different forms of estrogen becomes important. Yes, it's true that never carrying a biological pregnancy increases the risk of breast cancer by about 60 percent. The reason is quite interesting. Pregnancy increases the level of an estrogen called estriol, which is a more protective form of estrogen. This protective hormone is thought to cut your risk of breast cancer. So in this case, the risk factor is not something to which you actually expose your body—but rather, something to which you *don't* expose yourself. As you can see, risk factors work in many ways.

> Not sure. But here's one good thing—at least you won't have to watch Barney.

◆ WHAT IF I HAD MY FIRST PREGNANCY AT AGE THIRTY-SEVEN—DOES THIS INCREASE MY RISK OF BREAST CANCER?

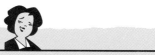

In general, the more pregnancies you carry to term, and the earlier in life you carry them, the greater the protection against breast cancer. On the flip side of that coin, the fewer pregnancies you carry, and the later you carry them, the greater your risk of breast cancer. One surprising statistic is this: 17 percent of breast cancer could be prevented if women had a full-term pregnancy by the age of twenty-five. Of course, our society is not moving in this direction—in fact,

> No, but it increases your chance of being fifty-seven when the child's twenty.

in many parts of this country and the world, women are having fewer children, and having them later in life. Over time, this may reveal itself in higher breast cancer rates.

Having your first child after the age of thirty produces a 40 percent greater risk of breast cancer than having your first child before age thirty. But remember, that 40 percent increase should be taken in proper context: since your basic risk of breast cancer at age thirty is 1 in 2,525, a 40 percent increase in risk means you'd now have a risk of 1 in 1,515—far from a certainty.

Fewer than 1 in 5 breast cancers are diagnosed in women under age forty, but we see more and more women in their forties getting pregnant. The result is that approximately 2 to 3 percent of women who are diagnosed with breast cancer will be diagnosed during pregnancy and lactation (breast-feeding). It appears that during the pregnancy itself, when the body is experiencing a rapid change in the estrogen balance—that is, the ratio of good and bad estrogens, plus other hormone changes—the breast is temporarily more vulnerable to cancer. Afterward, though, the experience of a full-term pregnancy creates a more stable, positive estrogen profile in the body, and cuts the long-term risk of breast cancer ten years after the pregnancy itself.

The issue of breast cancer treatment during pregnancy and lactation is covered on pages 179–82.

◆ DOES ABORTION, OR MISCARRIAGE, RAISE THE RISK OF BREAST CANCER?

Maybe, and maybe not. While many studies have found that there is no connection between spontaneous or induced abortion and the risk of breast cancer, there is some evidence that it does, in fact, increase a woman's risk, particularly if she has had no previous biological children. The theory is that the breast is more susceptible to cancer during the early stages of a pregnancy and shortly after delivery, when the breast cells are undergoing tremendous change and hormones in the body are fluctuating fast. These are considered "unstable," and therefore vulnerable phases for the body. The difference between an early pregnancy loss and a full-term pregnancy in terms of breast cancer risk may operate as follows: with an early pregnancy loss, you get only a short-term increased risk of breast cancer; with a full-term pregnancy, you get a short-term increased risk, followed by more important long-term protection against breast cancer.

◆ I'M TRYING TO DECIDE WHETHER TO BREAST-FEED MY BABY, AND I'VE READ THAT IN ADDITION TO BOOSTING MY CHILD'S HEALTH, THIS COULD HELP REDUCE MY RISK OF BREAST CANCER. SHOULD THIS PLAY INTO MY DECISION?

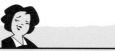

There is evidence that the longer and the earlier you breast-feed, the lower your risk of breast cancer. Most of this data is based on studies from other countries, since so few women in the U.S. breast-feed for long periods of time. There is some fascinating research on Tanka boat women from China, for example. These women wear a type of shirt that only opens on one side, forcing them to breast-feed only from one breast. Studies have shown that among this group of Chinese women, the suckled breast has a lower rate of cancer than the unsuckled one.

Yes, unless you want to wake up in the middle of the night and rinse out bottles.

Breast-feeding has been shown to lower the risk of breast cancer in younger, premenopausal women. And other research shows a possible relationship between breast-feeding and the baby's own risk of cancer: one report found that breast-feeding even for a short period of time can lower the risk of blood cancers (such as leukemia) in the breast-fed children.

There are several theories on how breast-feeding might protect women from breast cancer. One explanation involves the estrogen theme I keep talking about: that is, breast-feeding suppresses ovulation, and thereby cuts the body's exposure to estrogen. Another interesting theory is that breast-feeding mechanically cleanses the breast, removing unidentified contaminants, including carcinogens (cancer-causing agents) from the breast ducts. (Fortunately, babies cannot absorb all these contaminants early in life.) This theory is similar to one about colon cancer—i.e., that eating more fiber mechanically clears carcinogens from the colon, thereby lowering the risk of this type of cancer. Yet another hypothetical explanation is that breast-feeding lowers the risk of breast cancer by creating a beneficial pH balance in the breast. The *un*suckled breast creates an alkaline condition, which in turn predisposes to abnormal, precancerous conditions such as atypical hyperplasia in the breast. Finally, another theory holds that the failure to breast-feed successfully reflects some other underlying hormonal imbalance, which might predispose to cancer.

Whatever the reason, breast-feeding does seem to offer some protection against breast cancer in younger, premenopausal women. And since it is also the best source of nutrition for a growing baby, with countless emotional and health benefits (including a lowered risk of many infections, and better overall immunity), if it's possible for you to do it, it's a win-win for both you and your child.

◆ MY MOTHER AND GRANDMOTHER BOTH HAD BREAST CANCER. AM I GUARANTEED TO GET IT, TOO?

Happily, no. Your risk is higher than that of a woman with no family history, but you certainly aren't guaranteed of getting breast cancer. Many people with strong family histories of breast cancer perceive their risk of this disease to be greater than it actually is. In fact, only 5–10 percent of breast cancers develop because of inherited genetic defects (including such breast cancer genes as BRCA1,

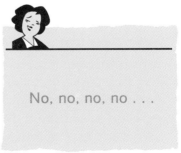

No, no, no, no . . .

BRCA2, p53, and ATM, among others). If your mother had breast cancer before she reached menopause, for example, your risk of getting breast cancer is two to three times higher over your entire lifetime—only a few percentage points higher than the rest of the general population. But if you have a first-degree relative (i.e., mother, daughter, or sister) who was diagnosed with premenopausal breast cancer in both breasts, the risk is much greater—nine times higher.

Everyone's personal and family breast cancer profile is different. This is why I recommend that my patients sit down with a genetic counselor to map out their personal situations, and try to ascertain their own risk of breast and other cancers based not only on their family history, but also their other possible risk factors (or protective factors) that have nothing to do with family history. You'd be surprised how detailed and customized the information can be. If you indeed find out that you are at relatively high risk of getting breast cancer, you, your doctor, and genetic counselor can design a screening regimen that's appropriate for you. This might involve an earlier-than-average first mammogram, more frequent breast examinations—or nothing out of the ordinary. In either case, putting some tangible advice in place of your great fear of this disease will only let you live more comfortably inside your own body.

◆ Do BIRTH CONTROL PILLS CAUSE BREAST CANCER?

The short answer is "very slightly, if at all." There is some evidence that oral contraceptives, or birth control pills, can increase the risk of breast cancer among certain groups of women. For example, women who took the older, higher-dose estrogen pills for many years, e.g., starting in their teens and into their thirties, seem to be at slightly greater risk of breast cancer compared to women who did not take that pill. According to a study by the U.S. Centers for Disease Control and Prevention and the American College of Obstetricians and Gynecologists, oral contraceptives add about 11 cancers per 100,000 women per year. On the other hand, older women who have taken the pill may have a *decreased* risk of breast cancer—this same report found that among older women who took the pill, there may be 18 *fewer* breast cancers per 100,000 women per year. When you bunch all age groups together, the possible increased breast cancer risk all but vanishes.

Interestingly, cancer diagnosed while women are on hormone replacement therapy tends to be caught earlier. This could be an inherent bias—that is, it could be due to the fact that these women are screened more carefully for breast cancer *because* they are taking hormone replacement therapy. Or, it's possible that tumors that develop under the influence of hormone replacement therapy are slower growing and "better behaved" than other cancers. This is just theory, however.

One thing I'm very leery about is comparing apples to oranges when it comes to the risk of breast cancer. It makes little sense to try to compare the lowest-dose estrogen pills many women are taking today to higher-dose older pills. Because the pill is an effective and efficient form of contraception, women should not be so quick to throw it out based on conflicting data. That said, however, there may be certain categories of women who are at greater risk than others—such as women who carry a gene for breast cancer, or those with strong family histories of the disease or other important risk factors. This is an issue you should take up with your own doctor, so that you can weigh the risks and benefits of pill use in your own personal case.

Remember that women carrying a mutation in either the BRCA1 or BRCA2 gene have an increased risk of *both* breast and ovarian cancer. Since oral contraceptives appear to *lower* the risk of ovarian cancer, it's entirely plausible that they could be beneficial to women in this group. But this needs further study.

Finally, on a related topic, two other hormonal contraceptives—progestin-only pills and Depo Provera (the long-lasting injectable progestin), although not as well studied as contraceptives containing estrogen—do *not* appear to increase breast cancer risk. However, the studies to date are somewhat limited and inconsistent, and further studies are needed to clarify these findings.

 ◆

◆ MY DOCTOR DIAGNOSED A PROBLEM IN MY BREASTS CALLED "ATYPICAL DUCT HYPERPLASIA." WILL THIS TURN INTO BREAST CANCER?

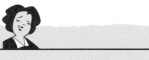

No, it will turn into a beautiful swan.

Not necessarily, but it can. Atypical duct hyperplasia is a precancerous condition that requires close supervision—but there is certainly no guarantee that it will progress into breast cancer. About 95 percent of so-called fibrocystic changes in the breast are not precancerous. This condition falls into the 5 percent category that can progress to cancer over time. Women with a family history of breast cancer who have this condition are more likely to develop breast cancer than those with no such family history. However, again, there are no guarantees that this will happen. To give you an idea of the percentages at stake here, atypical duct hyperplasia increases the risk of developing an invasive breast cancer by almost four and a half times. Add to this a first-degree relative with breast cancer (mother, sister, or daughter) and the risk increases to almost nine times that of other women.

It's very important that if you get a diagnosis of this condition by a needle biopsy, your doctor performs a follow-up surgical excision to be sure that cancer is not being overlooked in that breast. This is because sometimes cancers are found along with the precancerous condition—and also because the diagnosis of atypical duct hyperplasia itself can be misinterpreted. There is such a variety of potential findings—including a high number of normal cells, an unusual number of abnormal cells, and many other permutations on this theme—and some increase your risk of cancer. For this reason, it's very important to get a specific diagnosis (and prognosis) from your doctor, and a clear plan of future action. Ask your doctor for a copy of your pathology report and make sure you know what it means. This is *not* always given—or explained.

Just how carefully should you be followed up after this type of diagnosis? That depends. I do not believe in ordering mammograms every six months for every abnormal (but benign) finding. This is overkill. You might need more frequent physical examinations by your doctor, or more frequent mammograms for a select period of time. Talk to your doctor about what the best course of action is, taking into account your precise diagnosis and other possible risk factors as well.

Opposite, I've assembled a chart with the various non-cancerous breast changes, and the potential increased risk of breast cancer associated with each one. These foreign terms—in the language known as "medicalese"—may turn up on your pathology report, and it's important for you to know what they

Very heavy material here. Desperately needed song break:

To the tune of "Happy Days Are Here Again"

Happy boobs will grace your chest
If you go and get this simple test
I know that I am a major pest
(but!)
Mammograms are good for breasts.

It won't hurt, no not a bit
So avoid a premature obit
You're a little shy, who gives a . . . crap
Mammograms,
Mamm-o-grams,
Mammograms are good . . . that's it!

mean. This should help you to determine the real meaning of your breast cell changes, and whether or not you should be given special follow-up or treatment by your doctor:

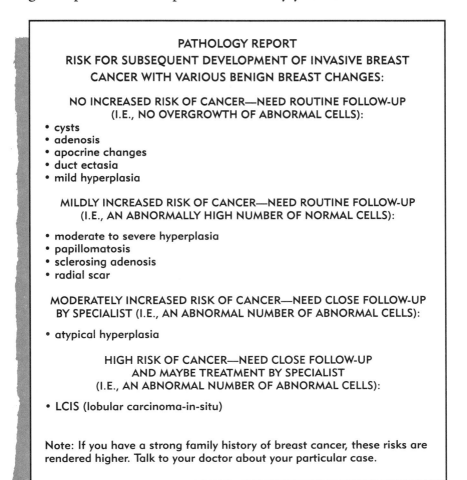

PATHOLOGY REPORT
RISK FOR SUBSEQUENT DEVELOPMENT OF INVASIVE BREAST
CANCER WITH VARIOUS BENIGN BREAST CHANGES:

NO INCREASED RISK OF CANCER—NEED ROUTINE FOLLOW-UP
(I.E., NO OVERGROWTH OF ABNORMAL CELLS):
- cysts
- adenosis
- apocrine changes
- duct ectasia
- mild hyperplasia

MILDLY INCREASED RISK OF CANCER—NEED ROUTINE FOLLOW-UP
(I.E., AN ABNORMALLY HIGH NUMBER OF NORMAL CELLS):
- moderate to severe hyperplasia
- papillomatosis
- sclerosing adenosis
- radial scar

MODERATELY INCREASED RISK OF CANCER—NEED CLOSE FOLLOW-UP
BY SPECIALIST (I.E., AN ABNORMAL NUMBER OF ABNORMAL CELLS):
- atypical hyperplasia

HIGH RISK OF CANCER—NEED CLOSE FOLLOW-UP
AND MAYBE TREATMENT BY SPECIALIST
(I.E., AN ABNORMAL NUMBER OF ABNORMAL CELLS):
- LCIS (lobular carcinoma-in-situ)

Note: If you have a strong family history of breast cancer, these risks are rendered higher. Talk to your doctor about your particular case.

To the tune of "YMCA"

Sister
You cannot live without—
I said sister—
It's dumb to go without—
I mean, sister—
It's what health is about—
There's no need to hide in fear and—

Ladies—
Get your squoosh and your squish
I said, ladies—
Serve 'em up on a dish—
Listen, ladies—
Set a time and I wish—
That you'd call your doctor be-cause—

Now is the time to get your mammogram—
So you can tell all your worries to scram—
Put your boobs to the test—
Get a load off your chest—
To pro-tect yourself get checked out—

Now is the time to get your mammogram—
For just a sec you might feel like canned ham—
And unlike root canal—
Here you can bring a pal—
Save your life, boobs, and your receipt—

Get this T-shirt!
Get this free shirt!—
(repeat, to end)

❖ CAN ANY SINGLE FOOD, OR TYPE OF DIET, PROMOTE— OR DETER—BREAST CANCER?

This is one of the most hotly controversial topics in breast cancer research today. Studies have produced different answers, and as a result you'll find "experts" strongly polarized on the subject of diet and its relationship to breast cancer. The most popular answer to your question is that a low-fat, high-fiber diet may—yes, *may*—reduce the risk of breast cancer. Many agree that the whole issue boils down—yet again—to the question of how much of the hormone estrogen is circulating in your body. Here's what I mean:

When you eat the typical American woman's diet, with about 38 percent of total calories from fat, you end up with lots of circulating estrogen. This diet, rich in the worst kind of fats—saturated animal fats, and junky fats from fried and packaged foods—promotes a whole host of diseases, including colon cancer and heart disease. Remember, animal fat can itself absorb toxic chemicals. Does it also promote breast cancer? That's the key question. Dr. David Rose and colleagues at the American Health Foundation believe that it does. They did a study in which they asked a group of women with typical high-fat American diets to change their food intake so that it would more closely resemble the lower-fat diet of women living in rural Japan. They chose this model because women in rural Japan have significantly lower breast cancer rates than women in the U.S. What they found was that after only three months, women who lowered their fat intake from 38 percent of total calories to 20 percent of total calories experienced a significant change in the levels of estrogen in their bodies. The more potent form of estrogen, called estradiol, and a milder form, called estrone, both dropped by 20 percent. This is believed by many researchers to be a significant enough drop to lower the risk of breast cancer. Subsequent studies have suggested that even lower fat intakes—at, say, 10–15 percent of total calories from fat—would be even better, even if it does knock some of the fun out of life. However, while this all makes excellent sense, no one has directly shown a reduction in breast cancer risk as a result of changed diet.

A similar pattern emerged when the researchers looked at the impact of a high-fiber diet on estrogen levels in the blood. Again, American women tend to have diets relatively poor in fiber (that is, foods like wheat and oat bran, and many vegetables, fruits, and grains). So they asked women who normally consumed just 15 grams of fiber per day to double their fiber intake—to 30 grams a day. This put their fiber intake at a level similar to women in rural Finland, another region where breast cancer levels are relatively low. Again, after just a few months, the women's circulating estrogen levels had dropped by about 20 percent. Dr. Rose found that the effective agent was wheat bran. But he and others believe that a more balanced increase in many types of high-fiber foods would still be the best approach in fighting breast cancer, as other high-fiber foods such as vegetables and fruits contain additional anticancer chemicals. Once again, no one has shown that a diet high in fiber can directly reduce the risk of breast cancer. But the powerful reduction in estrogen levels suggests such a benefit is possible.

So HOW DO I KEEP MY FAT INTAKE LOW ENOUGH, AND MY FIBER INTAKE HIGH ENOUGH, TO MAKE A DIFFERENCE IN MY HORMONES?

To lower fat intake that significantly you'd need to eliminate some of the biggest fat sources in the American diet. For example, switching from high-fat to nonfat dairy products would be a significant start. Nonfat milk, yogurt, and cheese are just as good for your bones as their fatty counterparts, but a lot easier on your weight, your heart—and estrogen levels. Fatty meats—including processed lunch meats—should be limited sharply. And all of those artificial, processed foods—like many packaged donuts, French fries, and so on—should be eaten only as rare treats. They are loaded with fat and have little else to recommend them. Trimming the fat off chicken, broiling instead of frying, using jam instead of butter—these kinds of wholesale shifts in the way you eat can make a huge dent in your total fat intake.

As for fiber, here's a look at the fiber content of various foods. This should give you a good idea of what it takes to consume 30 or more grams of fiber per day—and as you can see, it takes some doing. A fantastic start would be with some sort of bran cereal for breakfast in the morning or as a snack during the day, as these cereals have much more dietary fiber than other common foods.

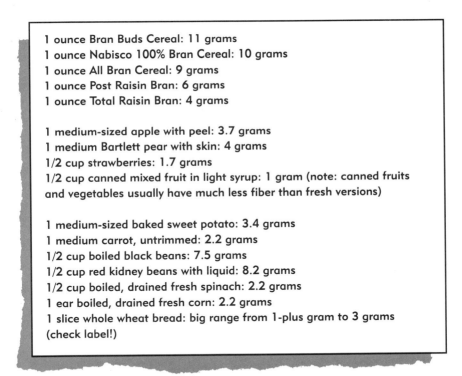

1 ounce Bran Buds Cereal: 11 grams
1 ounce Nabisco 100% Bran Cereal: 10 grams
1 ounce All Bran Cereal: 9 grams
1 ounce Post Raisin Bran: 6 grams
1 ounce Total Raisin Bran: 4 grams

1 medium-sized apple with peel: 3.7 grams
1 medium Bartlett pear with skin: 4 grams
1/2 cup strawberries: 1.7 grams
1/2 cup canned mixed fruit in light syrup: 1 gram (note: canned fruits and vegetables usually have much less fiber than fresh versions)

1 medium-sized baked sweet potato: 3.4 grams
1 medium carrot, untrimmed: 2.2 grams
1/2 cup boiled black beans: 7.5 grams
1/2 cup red kidney beans with liquid: 8.2 grams
1/2 cup boiled, drained fresh spinach: 2.2 grams
1 ear boiled, drained fresh corn: 2.2 grams
1 slice whole wheat bread: big range from 1-plus gram to 3 grams (check label!)

◆ WHY ALL THE HOOPLA ABOUT SOY-BASED FOODS FIGHTING BREAST CANCER?

Again, researchers have always been interested in learning why some populations have a lower risk of breast cancer than others—and diet is believed to play one part in the puzzle. Japanese women, who have much lower breast cancer rates than American women, eat large

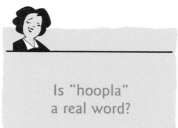

Is "hoopla" a real word?

amounts of soy-based foods. Soy-based foods, known as isoflavonoids, have received some attention of late not only for their potential impact on breast cancer risk, but also for their effects in mitigating some menopausal symptoms, such as hot flashes. Soy is a plant estrogen (called a phytoestrogen)—which might make you think it's a bad thing, since estrogen can fuel breast cancer. Soy contains genistein, which has been found to fight new blood vessel growth, which could, theoretically, starve a tumor. (There's a theory that eating lots of plant estrogen can trick the body into thinking it has received enough estrogen—satisfying the "hungry" estrogen receptors on cells—but in fact, only offering the benefits, and not the risks, of estrogen.) The same can be said of another group of foods known as lignans (high in fiber and omega-3 fatty acids), including flax seed (which I happen to adore and sprinkle liberally on my salads and oatmeal), rye, and sesame seeds. Like soy, lignans are also high in phytoestrogens. Chew flax seeds well to get all the benefits. The typical Japanese diet consists of 75 grams of soy protein daily. To give you an idea of just how much this is, 1½ cups of bean curd (firm variety) or three soy powder shakes is equivalent to 60 grams of soy protein.

Finally, cruciferous vegetables such as broccoli, cauliflower, cabbage, mustard greens, and Brussels sprouts contain a compound called indole-3-carbinol, which also has been shown to decrease the "bad" estrogen in the body. So when your grandmother told you to eat your greens, she was really ahead of her time. I urge my patients to do as I do and eat these foods on a regular basis.

◆ I'VE READ THAT ALCOHOL INCREASES THE RISK OF BREAST CANCER. HOW MUCH IS TOO MUCH?

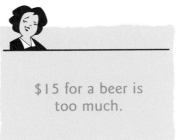

$15 for a beer is too much.

A number of studies have found a link between regular alcohol consumption and the risk of breast cancer. Although there is no completely satisfying biological explanation for how alcohol increases risk, one plausible theory is that alcohol increases estrogen levels in the body. In fact, there is evidence that the combination of drinking alcohol and taking hormone replacement therapy (i.e., estrogen) can be especially risky. Drinking alcohol while taking estrogen after menopause can raise the levels of estrogen in the body to about the point it reaches during ovulation! And the effect can last for hours after drinking is stopped.

How much is too much alcohol?

For women taking estrogen, even small amounts of alcohol—a half glass of wine per day—increase the risk of cancer nearly twofold. The greater the amount of alcohol, the greater the risk. Here are some more hard numbers for women *not* taking estrogen (though they vary from study to study): The risk of an invasive breast cancer is 41 percent higher among women who drink between 2 and 5 bottles of beer per day; between 2.8 and 5.6 glasses of wine per day; or between 2 and 4 shots of liquor per day. Three glasses of wine per day increases your risk of breast cancer by 30–40 percent. I often tell my patients to limit their alcohol consumption to two to three glasses of wine or other alcohol *per week*—if they choose to drink at all.

I'M CONSIDERING TAKING HORMONE REPLACEMENT THERAPY AFTER MENOPAUSE. WILL THIS INCREASE MY RISK OF BREAST CANCER?

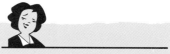

No, but it will increase your bill for hormone replacement.

This is an extremely tricky and controversial subject. When you look at fifty-one major studies about the impact of hormone replacement therapy on the risk of breast cancer, and take into consideration both current and recent users of hormone replacement, you find a 30 percent (i.e., modest) increase in the risk of breast cancer across the board. But this is a very broad-stroke way to look at the data, and it can be misleading for many women. For example, the degree of possible increased risk depends on various factors, including the following: (1) the duration of use of hormones; (2) how many years have passed since you stopped taking hormones (the risk seems to largely disappear after five years); (3) whether or not you took a break from the hormones at any point in your therapy; and (4) other factors. To make matters even more confusing, hormone replacement therapy is not one single thing; there are different formulations, including a major difference—some women take estrogen alone, while others take a combination of estrogen and a form of progesterone. Here is the old apples and oranges problem again.

The decision about whether to take hormone replacement therapy after menopause requires a careful evaluation of the seesaw balance among various risks and benefits for *you*. This risk-balance ratio will not be the same as it is for your best friend, your neighbor, or any other woman, for that matter. The first important question to ask yourself is why you are taking hormones. There are many reasons women choose to do so. On the benefit side, hormone replacement may offer protection against heart disease, which remains the number one killer of American women, though more women focus on—and fear—breast cancer than heart disease. Hormone replacement therapy also protects us from osteoporosis, the thinning of bone that can lead to fractures and permanent disability. And more recently, there is impressive data showing that hormone replacement therapy helps protect the brain against dementia so common in old age. Hormones also help stave off the disruptive symptoms of menopause, such as hot flashes, vaginal dryness and pain, mood changes, sleep problems, and so on. (Just to put things in some perspective, consider this: In the United States, a woman has a 23 percent lifetime risk of dying of heart disease, a 4 percent risk of dying of breast cancer, and a 2.5 percent risk of bone fractures from osteoporosis. The key is to work with your doctor to determine which, if any, of these risks is greater in your particular case—because of family history and other risk factors for these diseases.)

◆ So what's the bad news about estrogen therapy?

So far, I've discussed the protective qualities of estrogen. Of course, there is a downside as well. Estrogen, as we have heard again and again, may promote some kinds of cancers. We know that taking "unopposed" estrogen—that is, taking estrogen replacement therapy without progesterone—increases your risk of cancer of the lining of the uterus. And there is the possible increased risk of breast cancer among longtime users (although, as I said at the outset, this is a modest increased risk and depends on several variables). When you add a form of progesterone to the estrogen therapy, you erase the risk of cancer of the lining of the uterus. But you might also erase some of the protection against heart disease—which could be the most powerful reason for taking hormones. The effect of progesterone on breast cancer risk is still uncertain.

The story is a long and complex one, and impossible to cover in great detail in this small space. Some have even posed the important possibility that hormones might prolong life for women, thereby allowing them to live long enough to develop breast cancer they might not otherwise have lived to get! There

❖ ❖ ❖ ❖ ❖ ❖ ❖ ❖ ❖ ❖ ❖ ❖ ❖ ❖ ❖ ❖ ❖ ❖ ❖ ❖

are so many unresolved research issues. But there are a few bot-tom-line concepts to consider. If, for example, you have a strong family history of heart disease or stroke—your mother and father both died of heart attacks, for example—and you have other major risk factors for heart disease, including obe-sity, high blood pressure, high cholesterol, a sedentary lifestyle, diabetes, and so on—the scale for *you* might tip in *favor* of tak-ing hormones. On the other hand, if you have a personal his-tory of breast cancer, the scale will tip in favor of *not* taking hormones. Studies are now looking at the impact of hormone replacement for women with early, estrogen receptor–negative tumors with no evidence of disease after two years (or, when the estrogen status of the tumor is unknown, then no evidence of disease after ten years). I personally look forward to having some definitive data on the safety—or lack thereof—of hor-mone treatment in these women.

In addition to the potential increased risk of breast cancer, hormone therapy makes the breasts more dense—i.e., similar to younger women's breasts—and therefore difficult to study with mammography. Searching for a cancer on the mammo-gram of a woman taking hormone therapy has been likened to looking for a polar bear in a snowstorm: white on white.

The fundamental point I try to make to all my patients is that the only intelligent way to make a decision about hor-mone replacement therapy is to sit down with an experienced health care practitioner and map out a personal chart of risks and benefits. Sure, there are some women for whom I would not routinely recommend hormone replacement—for just one example, if you were diagnosed with breast cancer *while taking hormones*, I would tell you to stop the hormones. This is be-coming a terribly fuzzy arena as more women are surviving breast cancer and are postmenopausal. The issue requires a careful look at the individual woman and her risk of other health problems throughout later life, including her breast can-cer prognosis and symptoms of estrogen deficiency. If your doctor gives you a fast, pat answer (in favor of, or against, hor-mones) without a detailed explanation of your case, demand some good reasons—or look for a second opinion—before popping a pill or being denied its benefits.

◆ I AM CONSIDERABLY OVERWEIGHT. DOES THIS AFFECT MY BREAST CANCER RISK?

Yes. Women who are overweight (and taller, interestingly) are at increased risk of breast cancer. Studies show that obesity plays a more important role in the development of breast cancer among postmenopausal women than it does in younger women. Still, weight control is best started when you're young, not only because good habits are formed early, but because the breast cells are developing and changing more at this stage of life, and therefore any risk factor—obesity included—could have a more meaningful effect at this time.

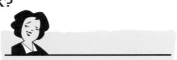

No, but stay away from horizontal stripes.

How is excess body weight related to the risk of breast cancer? There are several theories, but one brings us back to our old estrogen theme. Excess fat in the body boosts the amount of estrogen in the body, thereby potentially fueling the development of breast cancer. Another factor to consider is that not all body fat is the same. It seems that fat that settles in the middle of the body—on the belly and waist area—may be riskier than fat that settles on the buttocks or the legs. This middle-body fat, which often becomes more prominent after menopause, is associated not only with an adverse cholesterol profile and increased risk for diabetes, but also with higher estrogen levels. This could help explain the fact that increased weight in postmenopausal women is more predictive of breast cancer risk than it is in younger women. But again, much of this is still theoretical and under study.

Interestingly, weight gain is quite common after cancer treatment. More than half of premenopausal breast cancer survivors gain weight during the first postsurgical year. And women who undergo chemotherapy are prone to weight gain during treatment. Many women who undergo chemotherapy for early breast cancer gain an average of five to fourteen pounds; and 1 in 5 breast cancer survivors gains more than twenty pounds. Why? There are a few theories. First, the metabolic rate drops with chemotherapy. Second, many women decrease their physical activity during treatment, as a result of fatigue, depression, and malaise. Hormone treatments like tamoxifen (Nolvadex) and megestrol acetate (Megace) also can promote weight gain. If you find that your weight is spinning out of control during or after treatment, talk to your doctor and, ideally, sit down with a nutritionist with ample knowledge about breast cancer. This is not a time to try special diets you design yourself. You need the best nutrition possible to fight your disease and restore your energy. So don't make any big changes without expert advice.

♦ I CONFESS TO BEING A COUCH POTATO, AND I READ IN THE PAPER THAT THIS CAN INCREASE MY RISK OF GETTING BREAST CANCER. IS THERE ANY TRUTH TO THIS, OR IS THIS JUST PROPAGANDA FROM THE HEALTH POLICE?

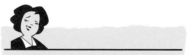

I'd answer your question, but I'm too busy to get off the couch. (And as far as I know, potatoes are good for you.)

Studies have shown that regular physical activity—exercise, that is—cuts your risk of breast cancer. The protection conferred by exercise seems to be greatest among younger, premenopausal women (under age forty-five), among lean women, and among those who have exercised regularly for at least three to five years. Regular exercisers have a 37 percent lower risk of breast cancer than sedentary women.

That said, what's the theory behind these findings? There are a number of interesting possibilities. For starters, physical activity may affect both the creation and excretion of hormones in the female body—and it may do so in a wide variety of ways. For instance, vigorous exercise among young women can cause a delay or pause in menstruation—which has been associated with a lowered risk of breast cancer. Exercise may also reduce obesity, especially fat in the middle, belly, or trunk of the body, which in turn would cut estrogen levels and the storage of contaminants attracted to fat. And there is a bit of data, albeit scarce, suggesting that the immune boost brought on by exercise is the protective factor.

Skeptics of the data linking exercise and breast cancer risk often argue that women who exercise have a number of *other* characteristics that put them at decreased risk of breast cancer, such as eating fewer calories, drinking less alcohol, eating less fat, and following other good lifestyle habits. Still, though, there is an increasing body of evidence supporting a role for exercise in the fight against breast cancer, even when studies control for other mitigating factors.

I urge my patients to exercise regularly—at least three to four hours per week—and vigorously if possible. I also practice what I preach. The bottom line is this: Physical activity will likely cut your risk of breast cancer, and it will definitely reduce your risk of other major killers like heart disease, stroke, diabetes, bone loss, and obesity. The benefits of regular exercise to overall physical and mental health cannot be overstated. While there is no magic bullet, no potion I can recommend to eradicate breast cancer and other major diseases that affect women, I do believe that exercise is up there with the most impressive ways to reduce your chance of disease and boost your chance of leading a healthy, vital life.

◆ ARE THERE AREAS IN THE COUNTRY WITH A HIGH INCIDENCE OF BREAST CANCER DUE TO PESTICIDES AND OTHER TOXINS?

Yes. For example, parts of Long Island, New York; Cape Cod, Massachusetts; the Great Lakes region; and San Francisco and

Los Angeles, California, are among a number of areas noted for higher than usual numbers of breast cancer cases. The reasons are unclear. In the case of Long Island, for example, it used to be common practice to spray pesticides all over farms and even suburban neighborhoods to help produce grow and lawns thrive. Agricultural uses stopped in the early 1970s, but by then hundreds of thousands of gallons of carcinogenic pesticides like DDT and other compounds had seeped into the shallow groundwater, and in turn got to work in women's bodies, promoting the risk of breast cancer. The theory goes as follows: DDT is what's known as a "xenoestrogen," a foreign estrogen compound that can raise levels of harmful estrogens in the human body. (There are good and bad xenoestrogens, as I discuss in other parts of this book. For instance, soy is a plant estrogen that may have some beneficial properties. See page 94.) When we are exposed to potentially *harmful* xenoestrogenic chemicals, our bodies convert the product into by-products or metabolites, which can pump up total estrogen levels in the body. Some studies have found that women with breast cancer from these areas have higher than normal levels of these compounds in

GEOGRAPHIC HOT SPOTS FOR BREAST CANCER IN THE U.S.

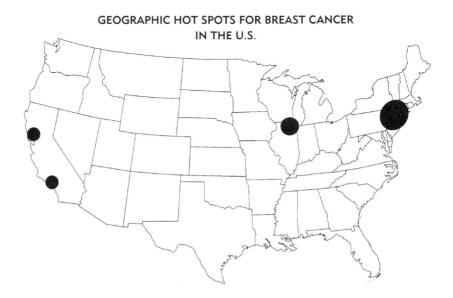

their blood. These metabolites linger in the fat of women's bodies for many years, raising the risk of breast cancer long after the spraying practice was stopped. And even though we no longer spray DDT in the United States for agriculture, we use many other compounds that also can change the body's hormone levels. And our use of lawn care products has soared—quadrupled within a decade in many areas. Plenty of third world countries continue to use DDT and many other xenoestrogens on their crops, so we may still be exposed to some of the effects of these pesticides when we eat foreign produce.

Studies are in progress examining the relationship of risk with other environmental agents (including toxic waste dumps, water contaminants, and air pollution).

So WHAT AM I SUPPOSED TO DO IF I HAVE BEEN EXPOSED TO A TOXIC ENVIRONMENT, OR GREW UP IN A "CANCER POCKET"?

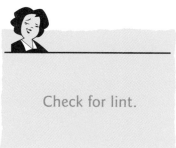

Check for lint.

The first thing to do is let your doctor know about your possible increased risk. Depending on your degree of exposure and on your general breast cancer risk profile, your doctor may want to be a little more vigilant about examining your breasts—perhaps more often than women without such chemical exposure.

Also keep in mind that if you are purchasing produce that has been exposed to pesticides of any kind (that is, nonorganic produce), you should very thoroughly wash the produce before eating it. There is a good deal of evidence that just rinsing water over your fruit is not adequate. Really scrubbing each item with soap and water, and sometimes peeling it, is likely needed to eliminate or at least greatly reduce the pesticide residue.

Should you be eating only organic fruits and vegetables? It's a nice idea, but not realistic—not to mention not affordable—for many people. Common sense tells me that it's worth being especially careful with young babies and girls going through puberty, as the breast cells are vulnerable and in flux at these times and may be more vulnerable to the effects of a variety of carcinogens, including pesticides. So maybe the mothers who feed their children organic produce aren't being overzealous.

The good news is things are better now than they were in the past. Hospitals, for example, have special methods of disposing of chemical waste, such as dioxane, mercury, and PVC (polyvinyl chloride); some carcinogenic chemicals, like those in the organochlorine family (i.e., DDT, DDE, and PCB), have been banned altogether; the government more closely regulates the use and disposal of chemicals on public property—and so on. The bottom line—use common sense. If a cleaning or garden product is clearly marked as dangerous for children, think about whether you want to expose *yourself* to much of it, either. Whenever possible, use natural products or avoid a product altogether.

Should you let the fear of cancer dominate your every thought and action? Certainly not. While there are some things we can do to reduce our risk, and lots we can do to catch cancers early, we cannot fully control our environment or the products to which we are exposed. Try not to allow your fears (even realistic fears) about cancer to darken your overall life experience. If you find that you are, in fact, obsessing over cancer avoidance, talk to your doctor or a counselor about your concerns.

QUESTIONS ABOUT THE INHERITED RISK OF BREAST CANCER:

◆ OF ALL THE RISK FACTORS FOR BREAST CANCER, ISN'T HEREDITARY RISK THE GREATEST?

It's hard to quantify and compare the impact of different risk factors, but in general, people greatly *overestimate* the power of genes to cause breast cancer. Certainly they are important, but not as much as most women believe. About 5–10 percent of breast cancers are thought to be due to an inherited predisposition. That leaves a whopping 90–95 percent that are not.

✦ WHAT EXACTLY ARE THE BRCA1 AND BRCA2 GENES?

Many people assume that these genes actually cause cancer. In fact, they are known as tumor-suppressor genes, which means that they act as *brakes* on cell growth, thereby reducing the risk of cancer. It is a *change* or mutation in these genes that increases one's risk of getting breast cancer. (These genes also predispose to ovarian and colon cancers in women, and to prostate, colon, and breast cancer in men.) However, having a mutation in one of these genes does not mean that you will definitely get cancer (more below). And just because one of your parents carries a mutated breast cancer predisposition gene, you aren't guaranteed to inherit it yourself. If you have a parent with a mutation, you have a 50 percent chance of inheriting the mutation yourself (I always urge patients to look at the glass half full: this also means that you have a 50 percent chance of *not* inheriting this mutation). And it's critical to remember that having the genetic mutation does not mean you absolutely will get cancer.

✦ SO WHAT'S THE RISK OF GETTING BREAST CANCER IF YOU CARRY ONE OF THESE GENES?

Research is still ongoing to determine the true answer to this question. But let me put this issue in context. First of all, the average woman has a *lifetime* breast cancer risk of 10–12 percent. This is a woman's risk of getting breast cancer by the time she reaches old age. If she carries a BRCA1 or BRCA2 gene mutation, her lifetime risk of breast cancer can go as high as 84 percent—but may be closer to 60 percent, research suggests.

✦ HOW CAN I FIND OUT IF I'M A CARRIER OF BRCA1 OR 2?

The process involves a blood test or, in some cases, a test of stored tissue samples, and is called "genetic testing." However, it's very important to undergo genetic counseling before jumping into the test. Genetic counseling involves a sit-down session of up to two hours in length—and sometimes more than one session—with a genetic counselor who is specially trained in the area of cancer genetics. The genetic counselor will take a detailed history of your own and your family's medical histories, and discuss your risk of developing cancer, as well as the benefits and limitations of genetic testing. To find a genetic counselor in your area who specializes in cancer genetics, call the National Society of Genetic Counselors. If you do opt to be tested for a breast cancer gene, the process usually takes several weeks and can cost up to $2,400. The cost is covered by some, but not all, insurers. There are also research studies in various parts of the country that can provide free testing to those who participate. Be sure to speak with the counselor about steps that can be taken to ensure your confidentiality.

◆ **IS IT TRUE THAT JEWISH PEOPLE ARE AT GREATER RISK OF CARRYING THESE RISKY BREAST CANCER GENES?**

People whose ancestors hail from central or eastern Europe and are of Ashkenazi Jewish background are at increased risk of carrying three particular mutations in either BRCA1 or BRCA2. These mutations occur in about 2.5 percent of Ashkenazi Jews, which is a much higher percentage than the estimated frequency of all mutations in BRCA1 and BRCA2 in the population at large. Because of this predisposition, Ashkenazi Jews who opt to undergo genetic testing are usually tested for these three mutations first. The cost is about $400–$500, and the results take about three to five weeks.

◆ **WHAT SHOULD I DO IF I CARRY ONE OF THESE "BREAST CANCER GENES"?**

If you're a woman, you should be vigilantly screened for breast, ovarian, and colon cancers. For breast cancer screening, do monthly breast self-examinations (see pages 64–72); have a regular physical examination of your breasts by your doctor (at intervals specified for your case); and have regular mammo-grams (again, let your doctor determine the best starting age and frequency for your case, as there is a theoretical concern that some young women with a genetic predisposition to breast cancer could be especially sensitive to radiation). For ovarian cancer screening, have a blood test called CA-125 (it's useful but not a perfect test); pelvic examinations by your doctor; and transvaginal ultrasound testing. Some centers use so-called Doppler technology (which studies blood flow through the ovaries) along with transvaginal ultrasound testing to increase this test's ability to catch cancers. Prophylactic (preventive) mastectomies and oophorectomy (removal of the ovaries) are also options considered by some women. And for colon cancer screening, have digital rectal exams by your doctor; fecal occult blood testing (in which your stool is tested for blood that can't be seen by the naked eye); and either sigmoidoscopy or colonoscopy. Again, for all of these tests, ask your doctor what the proper starting age and frequency of tests should be in your particular case.

If you're a man, you should be carefully screened for colon cancer (the same tests are used on women and men) and for prostate cancer. Prostate screening involves the digital rectal exam as well as a blood test for PSA, or prostate specific anti-gen. Recent research has suggested that the so-called free PSA blood test may be an even more effective predictor of prostate cancer than the traditional PSA test.

◆ MY MOTHER GOT PREMENOPAUSAL BREAST CANCER AT THE AGE OF FORTY. I'VE HEARD THIS PUTS ME AT EXTREMELY HIGH RISK OF THE DISEASE. TRUE?

I hear this question all the time, and almost every woman with this family history is shocked—and pleased—to learn that she has greatly overestimated her risk. You probably think you are guaranteed—or nearly assured—of getting breast cancer. In fact, your risk of getting breast cancer is only about 15–20 per-cent over your lifetime—just a few percentage points higher than that of the average woman. Now, take advantage of your knowledge and concern about breast cancer: follow the breast cancer screening guidelines discussed in chapter 2, talk to your doctor about the possibility of genetic counseling and about any special precautions that might be recommended in your case, and pay attention to the avoidable risk factors discussed throughout this chapter. A family history of breast cancer is no death sentence. Use the information as an opportunity to protect yourself and, perhaps someday, your own children as well.

◆ IS IT LEGAL FOR MY HEALTH BENEFIT PLAN TO DISCRIMINATE IN PROVIDING COVERAGE BASED ON GENETIC INFORMATION?

No, it is not legal. Health plans can refuse coverage based on certain pre-existing conditions—that is, diagnosed, clinical health problems. But carrying a mutation in a breast cancer predisposition gene—BRCA1 or 2, let's say—is not a health condition in itself. A federal law known as the Health Insurance Portability and Accountability Act of 1996 offers some protection against insurance bias related to genetic information; however, it only applies to people with group insurance. Different states have various laws related to this issue. Now let's say, on the other hand, that you have been diagnosed with breast cancer—that's a different story. Breast cancer could be considered a pre-existing condition and therefore legally subject to temporary limitations on coverage. Generally, the maximum period for exclusion from coverage is eighteen months, and in most cases "credit" must be given to reduce the exclusionary period when you change plans within two months.

If you have a legal problem related to genetic information, there are various advocacy groups which can help you navigate the system. See page 276 in the Resources section for details on how to contact them.

◆ CAN I PREVENT BREAST CANCER BY HAVING BOTH OF MY BREASTS REMOVED?

The answer is 90 percent yes—you'll cut your risk of breast cancer by 90 percent or even more if you have both breasts surgically removed. Breast cancer can appear in small amounts just under breast skin that is not surgically removed—which accounts for the remaining 10 percent risk. But what a high price to pay!

The procedure you're asking about is called "prophylactic mastectomy." It includes the removal of the nipple, the tissue surrounding the nipple known as the areola, and the underlying breast tissue. Breast reconstruction by a plastic surgeon is usually done immediately following the mastectomy.

Prophylactic or preventive mastectomy is done extremely rarely, but has been offered to the following women:

1. Those with a strong family or personal history of breast cancer;
2. Those with multiple previous breast biopsies that contained precancerous cells;
3. Those whose breasts are difficult to screen because (a) they have dense breast tissue, or (b) they have extremely lumpy breast tissue; and
4. Those with a severe fear of cancer—"cancerphobia."

Nowadays, most women who undergo this preventive surgery are carriers of the BRCA1 or BRCA2 cancer gene mutations. If you are considering taking this extreme measure to protect your health, be sure to educate yourself fully about your risk of cancer, and the risks of surgery, before making the move. This is a serious decision that deserves the utmost thought and preparation. That said, I must tell you that studies have shown that women who make this decision after careful, thorough consideration are generally pleased with the results.

BREAST CANCER RISK— AND RISK REDUCTION

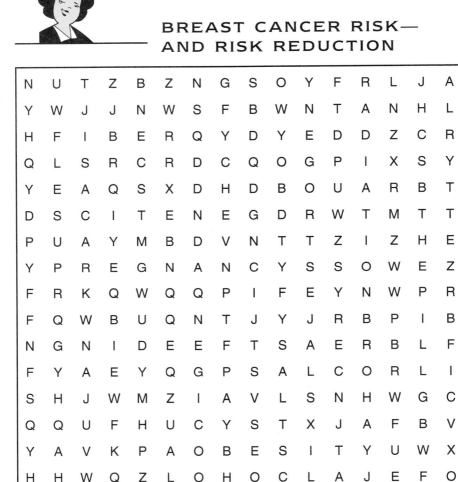

```
N  U  T  Z  B  Z  N  G  S  O  Y  F  R  L  J  A
Y  W  J  J  N  W  S  F  B  W  N  T  A  N  H  L
H  F  I  B  E  R  Q  Y  D  Y  E  D  D  Z  C  R
Q  L  S  R  C  R  D  C  Q  O  G  P  I  X  S  Y
Y  E  A  Q  S  X  D  H  D  B  O  U  A  R  B  T
D  S  C  I  T  E  N  E  G  D  R  W  T  M  T  T
P  U  A  Y  M  B  D  V  N  T  T  Z  I  Z  H  E
Y  P  R  E  G  N  A  N  C  Y  S  S  O  W  E  Z
F  R  K  Q  W  Q  Q  P  I  F  E  Y  N  W  P  R
F  Q  W  B  U  Q  N  T  J  Y  J  R  B  P  I  B
N  G  N  I  D  E  E  F  T  S  A  E  R  B  L  F
F  Y  A  E  Y  Q  G  P  S  A  L  C  O  R  L  I
S  H  J  W  M  Z  I  A  V  L  S  N  H  W  G  C
Q  Q  U  F  H  U  C  Y  S  T  X  J  A  F  B  V
Y  A  V  K  P  A  O  B  E  S  I  T  Y  U  W  X
H  H  W  Q  Z  L  O  H  O  C  L  A  J  E  F  O
```

Find and circle the following words:

ALCOHOL	FIBER	PREGNANCY
BREAST-FEEDING	GENETICS	RADIATION
DES	OBESITY	THE PILL
ESTROGEN		

4

WAKE-UP CALL:
The Breast Cancer Diagnosis

KATE JACKSON

After I had breast cancer, I wasn't the same. I've always counted on my body to do what I needed it to do, whether it be up sixteen hours in front of a camera or play tennis or run a mile. Whatever my body needed to do—I've always counted on it to do it. And suddenly, my body, this thing that's mine and only mine and me, I couldn't count on it. Because I had this breast cancer, I lost my personality, my faith in my body for years. Having breast cancer just blew me away. It was such a shock to my system, to my mind, to my body, to my everything. I felt that I just wasn't "me." I was just sort of a shell.

I don't really know how to explain it except to say that my whole personality went away. I spoke softly, and for the longest time I wouldn't go anywhere because stick me with somebody I didn't know, I couldn't say anything. You just walk around feeling that you must look as if you're in shock. You think that your lips must look white and you must look pale, you just must look as if you're about to faint all the time. You can't think. You can't even make small talk. I was shaken to the core.

I have to admit that after the lumpectomy, I somehow knew that my battle with breast cancer wasn't over. After I had it the second time, I thought it was over. I still think it is. Of course, there are always some days that I think it's not over. Nobody is a superwoman who gets it taken care of boom, done, and never thinks about it. I mean that's all a bunch of bullsh—.

So my message is this: Early detection is the key to the cure. Someday they'll be able to cure breast cancer, but for now, that's the best bet. I'm glad I've spoken out. Now that people are talking about it, people are becoming more aware and less frightened, and it's becoming less of a stigma. It was just a horrible stigma for women for so many years, and now the attitude has changed. Now it's "I'm a woman, I'm entitled to a life, I'm going to protect myself against breast cancer!"

◆ How long does it take for breast cancer to become detectable?

Quite a long time. Breast cancer cells take up to ten years to develop into a tumor that can be seen on a mammogram (breast X ray). And they take a few more years than that to become what's known as a "palpable mass"—that is, something your doctor can feel during a physical examination of your breast, or you can feel yourself. To give you an idea of why it takes this much time, consider this: a single breast cancer cell doubles every three months, on average. So after three months, there are two cells; after six months, there are four cells; after nine months, eight cells, and so on. After ten years, a breast tumor is about one centimeter in size—about the size of your pinky nail. This is about the smallest size at which your doctor can actually feel the mass during a physical examination of your breast, or you can feel it yourself.

Of course, one centimeter is an average. The important thing to remember is just how critical it is to have regular mammograms to detect breast cancer as early as possible. A mammogram can catch a breast cancer when it's no larger than a pencil point, whereas you might not feel a breast lump yourself until it reaches a full inch in size. But the test is not foolproof. About 20 percent of all breast cancers are not detected through routine screening mammography, and some are missed because of interpretational error or pure oversight. This should send home just how important it is to have a mammogram done at an accredited mammography facility every single year from age forty onward (or earlier if your doctor recommends it for your particular case). Regularity helps ensure that something missed one year will be caught the next.

◆ Is there any test that can catch breast cancer even before a mammogram can show it?

As of today, mammography is the best test for catching breast cancer in its so-called preclinical phase—that is, the period be-

TUMOR GROWTH RATE

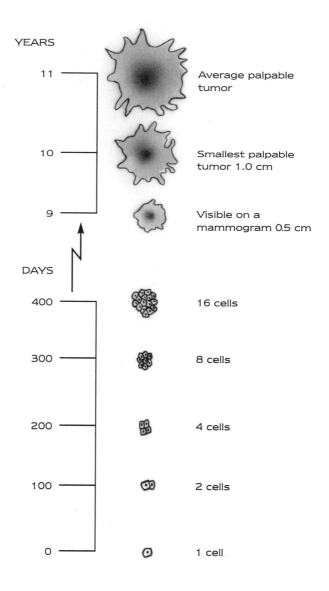

YEARS

11 — Average palpable tumor

10 — Smallest palpable tumor 1.0 cm

9 — Visible on a mammogram 0.5 cm

DAYS

400 — 16 cells

300 — 8 cells

200 — 4 cells

100 — 2 cells

0 — 1 cell

GOOD THINGS ABOUT DISCOVERING YOU HAVE BREAST CANCER:

1. Suddenly, lumps in the mashed potatoes aren't that upsetting.

2. You'll probably get to spend a lot more quality time getting to know your friendly insurance provider.

3. You have the perfect excuse not to attend your obnoxious nephew's piano recital.

4. Your husband probably won't mind mowing the lawn and washing the dishes.

5. If you've always hated your hair, good news, you'll probably be getting rid of it.

6. When people say, "What's wrong with you?" you can say, "Cancer," and then watch their faces turn white.

fore anyone, even your doctor, can feel it. Someday we hope to develop even better tests, such as a blood test that will detect cancers that consist of perhaps just a tiny group of cells. In the meanwhile, though, mammography is an excellent tool that saves thousands of lives every year—for both younger and older women. (For a chart on who should have mammograms and how often, see pages 52–53.) So the next time you feel lazy about going for your mammogram, remember that critical several-year period during which the mammogram can "see" a breast cancer, but no one can feel it. Take advantage of this potentially lifesaving window of opportunity.

◆ WHAT'S A BREAST BIOPSY AND HOW IS IT DONE?

A breast biopsy is a procedure in which your doctor takes a small sample of tissue or cells from your breast to see if the cells are benign (normal) or cancerous. There are several different ways to do a breast biopsy, depending on several factors, including whether the worrisome breast mass was actually *felt* by your doctor, or can only be detected on a mammogram (or some other imaging test). If your doctor can feel the mass, then he or she can do a biopsy without the aid of any special imaging tool. If the mass is only visible on a mammogram, for example, then your doctor will need to do the biopsy under the guidance of a special type of mammography machine, in order to guide the needle to the right location.

There are two main ways to harvest cells from the breast: (1) with a very thin needle, known as a "fine needle biopsy," which takes cells from the breast, and (2) with a larger needle, known as a "core needle biopsy," which takes a bit more tissue from the breast. When a fine needle biopsy is done, a specialized cell-reader known as a cytologist is needed to determine if the cells are cancerous or not. When a core needle biopsy is done, someone with less specialized training—a general pathologist—is able to "read" the tissue to determine its status.

One of the benefits of the fine needle biopsy is that it can be done quickly in the doctor's office with little preparation, little discomfort, and no local anesthesia. I often do this procedure (or a core procedure) in my office immediately after feeling a suspicious lump in my patient's breast, rather than scheduling a separate follow-up appointment for the biopsy. In addition, I often use the thin needle when I find a mass in the breast that I suspect could be a fluid-filled cyst and not a solid tumor. I insert the thin needle into the mass, and if fluid comes out, we can all rest easy. If there is no fluid, I will go on to perform a biopsy so that the cells can be checked for cancer. One downside to fine needle biopsy, however, is the fact that because just a few cells are gathered during the procedure, your doctor cannot tell if a cancer has invaded neighboring breast

I feel two songs coming on:

**Sung by Rosie and Olivia Newton-John
to the tune of "Physical"**

ROSIE: We're talkin' to the women over thirty-five
OLIVIA: You're doin' self-examination
ROSIE: We got another thing to keep you alive
Give your boobs a squeeze
OLIVIA: A mammogram makes sure that you have healthy breasts
ROSIE: No different than a cold waffle iron
OLIVIA: It reminds me of having my pants pressed
ROSIE: So make your move and please . . .
BOTH: Get a physical
Physical
Call and get a physical
Schedule a physical
Get yourself a mammogram
You'll thank us, ma'am
Get yourself a mammogram!
OLIVIA: You can do it, 'cause you're strong
It only hurts for five seconds
ROSIE: Whether they're tiny, big, or long
You know what they need . . .
OLIVIA: If you feel a marble, pea, or other flaw
Don't be shy, just get it checked
ROSIE: Be a trendsetter, just whip off your bra
Start a health stampede
BOTH: Get a physical
Physical
It's time for your physical
Don't say you're too busy-cal
Get yourself a mammogram
You'll thank us, ma'am
Get yourself a mammogram!

To the tune of "The Hokey Pokey"

You put your left breast in—
You take your left breast out—
You put your right breast in—
And they squoosh it all about—
Call now—make an appointment—
You'll be happy as a clam—
When you get a mammogram!

Hey!
You're over forty years—
And you got lotsa fears—
But when you get checked out—
All your worries disappear—
Your boobies need attention—
Why not give yourself a hand—
And go get a mammogram!

Hey!
I'll tell you all month long—
Avoiding it is wrong—
Because detection is—
The best way to keep you strong—
You know the subject's bigger—
Than McGwire's best grand slam—
So go get a mammogram!

tissue. The core needle biopsy, on the other hand, is a slightly more invasive procedure requiring local anesthesia. On the plus side, the core biopsy gives more information about the cancer cells' "architecture" and whether they have invaded neighboring breast tissue. Needle biopsies offer a number of benefits to patients: you don't need to miss a day of work, there are no pre-operative blood tests, no need to be picked up after the procedure, no scar tissue created (which can interfere with future mammograms), and no incision.

With any kind of breast biopsy, if the result is "positive"—that is, if it detects cancer cells—the results are almost certainly accurate. However, because fine needle biopsy takes just a few cells, there is a higher risk of "false negatives" with this procedure than there is with core biopsies—meaning that fine needle biopsy may miss a cancer that is actually there. It's easy to imagine why this might happen—you can liken it to fishing with a skinny line instead of with a net. Tiny cancers, or tumors that are very deep, mobile, or bloody are the easiest to miss. Core needle biopsy is less likely to make these errors.

One approach that helps me and my colleagues to reduce the risk of false negatives significantly is what we call the "triple diagnosis"—that is, the correlation (or lack thereof) among (1) the mammogram (if it shows anything), (2) what we can feel during a physical examination of the breast, and (3) the cell findings. When all of the pieces of the puzzle are put together, it is much easier to make a correct diagnosis. This is just one of many reasons why it is so very critical for (1) your radiologist, (2) your breast surgeon, and (3) your pathologist to communicate effectively.

◆ CAN A BIOPSY BE DONE ON A LUMP YOUR DOCTOR CAN'T FEEL?

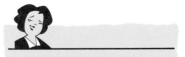

Sometimes you feel like a lump, sometimes you don't.

Yes. Your doctor will use the guidance of a mammography machine when doing a biopsy on a "nonpalpable mass" (one that can't be felt). It is possible to use a fine needle, core needle, or even a thicker needle in procedures known as the "Mammotome" or the "ABBI technique" (for Advanced Breast Biopsy Imaging technique). These image-guided biopsies are collectively known as "stereotactic biopsies." If the larger needle is required, I personally prefer the Mammotome method to the ABBI. As in so many areas of breast cancer care—and so many areas of medicine in general—there is a turf issue involved here. The question is, should these procedures be done by radiologists, or by surgeons. The radiologists are concerned that surgeons lack adequate skill in breast imaging; and the surgeons worry that the radiologists have never done breast biopsies and lack experience discussing breast cancer treatment options with patients. So to whom do these procedures belong? I feel strongly that it has to be a team effort in order to be most effective. When surgeons and radiologists work together performing and interpreting these image-guided needle procedures, the results improve significantly.

Another group of breast biopsies, known as surgical biopsies, is likely going the way of the dinosaur, thanks to the effec-

Different Types of Breast Biopsies

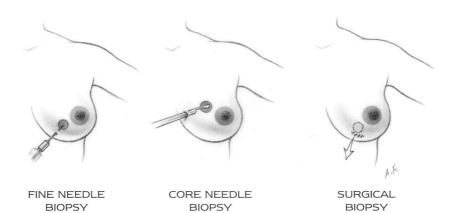

FINE NEEDLE   CORE NEEDLE   SURGICAL
BIOPSY   BIOPSY   BIOPSY

tiveness of the less-invasive needle procedures. One of these, called the "incisional biopsy," was often used on very large tumors in the past. Today, this type of biopsy has largely been replaced by the core biopsy, which offers the benefits of gathering a good amount of tissue without making an unnecessary trip to the operating room. Another is called the "excisional biopsy," in which the entire lesion is removed—but not necessarily with any surrounding breast tissue. The excisional biopsy has largely been replaced by the lumpectomy procedure, in which the whole tumor is removed *along with* a rim of normal surrounding tissue.

However, I always like to say that "a fool with a tool is still a fool"; just because needle biopsies are relatively easy to do and quite effective doesn't mean that they should be used willy-nilly on every lump in your breasts. If a biopsy is not needed, it is not needed, and women should not be put through any unnecessary procedure even if it's a relatively noninvasive one.

A final note: The handling of the breast cells is very important when it comes to getting an accurate biopsy result. I work with a nurse who is specially trained to process the cells in the right way, both air-drying them *and* using a fixative on glass slides. If the cells are not handled properly, it is possible to get false results even if the biopsy goes perfectly well and adequate cells are gathered. So I take this last step very seriously. You might want to ask your doctor if he or she takes special steps to ensure the quality of your harvested cells.

◆ WHY WOULD MY DOCTOR CHOOSE TO DO A BREAST BIOPSY?

If your doctor sees something suspicious on your mammogram—or feels something abnormal during the physical examination of your breast—or both—there are two possible courses of action. One, your doctor may do a biopsy then and there to determine if the mass

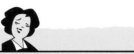

To impress his mom who scrubbed floors to put him through medical school.

is just a cyst, or something more serious. Second, if your doctor is unsure about whether the mass really is worrisome, you may be told to come back in a couple of months—after one or two menstrual cycles, for example. Or, if you happen to be taking birth control pills or postmenopausal hormone therapy, you may be asked to discontinue the use of the product for a couple of months and then brought back for a follow-up breast examination. Your doctor may also order a mammogram or other breast imaging tests, depending on your age.

◆ I KEEP HEARING THE TERM "MICROCALCIFICATIONS" IN THE BREAST? WHAT ARE THEY?

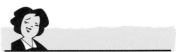

You shouldn't be hearing anything in your breasts.

Microcalcifications are little bits of calcium in the breast. For the most part (85 percent of the time) they are benign, harmless so-called fibrocystic changes in the breast. Microcalcifications show up as little white dots on a mammogram. They can be as small as a pencil point. We tend to worry about them when they appear in certain patterns—for instance, when five or more microcalcifications are found in a group; when they appear in a variety of sizes and shapes; when they are arranged in a line along a breast duct; and when they are associated with a breast mass. There are several theories as to where they originate, including the possibility that they represent debris from cell turnover in the breast; that cancer cells produce the calcium; and that they may develop after previous breast surgery or radiation. Also, we sometimes see a condition in which calcium literally floats inside benign cysts in the breasts, known as "milk of calcium" or "calcium in teacups." (Microcalcifications are *not*, as some people assume, caused by eating excessive dairy products.)

When microcalcifications are suspicious, we do a breast biopsy to determine whether cancer is involved. The (sterotactic)

core biopsy discussed earlier in this chapter is the a good way to
biopsy microcalcifications. I personally prefer even a thicker
needle in some cases, so I use the image-guided Mammotome
method for these biopsies.

◈ ARE THERE RISKS TO NEEDLE BIOPSIES?

With all types of needle biopsies, there is a very small but real
risk of bleeding, infection, injury to the underlying chest wall,
and getting unwanted air into the chest. The risk is, *theoretically*, slightly higher with the core needle than with the fine
needle, because more tissue is taken from the breast. But I'm
pleased to report that I have had *exceedingly* rare problems with
either procedure. Ask your doctor about his or her record and
experience.

Some women want to know if the needle biopsy itself
could dislodge cancer cells and spread them. The answer, again,
is *theoretically* yes—any disruption of the tissue in or around a
cancer could potentially jostle the cells and set them loose.

To be on the safe side, however, I use a technique that may
help reduce the risk of spreading cancer cells. When I take out
the site of the core of the cancerous tissue, I also take out a
small piece of the skin that surrounds the needle's entrance
point into the breast, along with what's known as the "needle
tract"—that is, the area through which the core needle is
dragged to pull out the cancer cells. You can think of this as
similar to wiping away footprints from the scene of a crime.
You might want to ask your doctor whether he or she does this
as well.

The important thing for every woman to know is that
there is NO change in survival rates among women who have
had needle biopsies followed by breast cancer surgery, versus
those who had no biopsy and went straight to surgery. This
means that regardless of whether a couple of breast cancer cells
are dislodged during a needle biopsy, there is no resulting impact on your prognosis. And since the needle biopsy can offer
critical information to guide your surgeon, it is quite valuable.

◆ WHAT TOOLS ARE USED TO DIAGNOSE BREAST CANCER, AND WHY MIGHT MY DOCTOR CHOOSE ONE OVER ANOTHER?

The best, most sensitive test for the diagnosis of breast cancer is the mammogram, or breast X ray. However, there are several other tests that have their place in our diagnostic arsenal. The following imaging tools are to be used in addition to—not instead of—mammography. They may help to reduce the number of unnecessary biopsies; aid in the early detection of breast cancer in certain groups of women who are harder to examine (due to very lumpy breast tissue) or to study with mammograms (as a result of very dense breast tissue or because of previous radiation treatment, or multiple previous biopsies); to investigate the status of breast implants; and other special cases.

• **SONOGRAMS:** The sonogram is a test with no radiation that involves bouncing sound waves off a shape or structure, creating an image we can read on a screen. When the sonogram is used to image the breast, it tends to pick up lots of masses that are not cancer—such as cysts and other benign lumps. In the past, sonograms were mainly used to offer backup information after a mammogram picked up something suspicious. These days, however, sonography is being targeted to certain groups of women for whom mammography can be trickier—such as young women with very dense breast tissue, women with extremely lumpy breasts, and women with strong family histories of breast cancer. Sonograms are very operator-dependent and more time-consuming than mammography; there is a steep learning curve, so it helps to have someone with experience reading the results. Its main role is, and should be, as an *adjunct* to mammography in certain groups of women—not yet as a primary screening test on its own.

• **MRI:** Magnetic resonance imaging or MRI is also being touted as useful in women with dense breasts and those with a strong family history of breast cancer. The high-resolution images offered by this test have proved helpful in determining the extent of early breast cancers of a type known as DCIS—or ductal carcinoma-in-situ (cancers limited to breast ducts). A diagnosis of cancer on MRI is likely to be accurate. But as with the sonogram, the *failure* to detect cancer with MRI is *not* a guarantee that you are cancer-free.

• **PET scans:** Positron emission tomography or PET scans are also being studied as a possible tool to screen women with very dense breast tissue. However, this test has another potentially exciting use as well. It seems that PET scans might help determine how well the most advanced cancers are responding to chemotherapy or other cancer treatments. The PET scan response may precede any clinical improvement—letting doctors and patients know, early on, how well they're doing, or if treatment needs to change.

• **SESTAMIBI scan:** This test, also called the technetium Tc 99m Sestamibi (Miraluma) scan, involves a radioactive material for use in studying breasts that are tough to image with other standard tools. Still only under scientific study to determine its benefits in breast cancer diagnosis, this tool has been in use for over a decade to examine the heart. As with MRI, a diagnosis of cancer on the Sestamibi scan is likely to be accurate, but a *failure* to detect cancer with this method is *not* reliable.

◆ WHO DIAGNOSES BREAST CANCER?

Most breast cancers are initially picked up by the primary care provider—whether that person is a general physician, a gynecologist, a nurse practitioner, or some other general medical care provider. If something suspicious is found, however, it is important

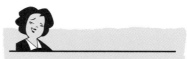

Marcus Welby, Doug Ross, Dr. Seuss, Dr. Ruth, Dr. Strangelove.

to be seen by a surgeon with experience in breast disease. You might be surprised to learn that there is no special board certification for becoming a breast surgeon. This means, unfortunately, that there are a lot of self-proclaimed breast surgeons running around who might not, in fact, have special expertise in the area. If you want to find a good breast surgeon to confirm a diagnosis of breast cancer, your best bet is to find someone who is a board certified surgeon, and who attends special courses and conferences on surgery of the breast. It would also be wise to find someone who is a fellow of the American College of Surgeons, which would indicate that he or she has done a minimum number of procedures in the field and has proven some level of expertise to his or her peers. If you can find someone who focuses only on breast surgery, all the better—specialization helps ensure experience. But certainly there are good breast surgeons out there who do other types of operations as well. The American College of Surgeons, based in Chicago, puts out a very useful pamphlet on how to interview your potential surgeon.

It's also somewhat reassuring if your surgeon has been recertified (now required every ten years by the American Board of Surgery).

Finally, in coming up with a definitive diagnosis (and then treatment plan) of breast cancer, it is valuable to have a team of experts working in concert. For example, your breast surgeon, a radiologist who specializes in breast imaging, a radiation oncologist, a plastic surgeon if need be, a medical oncologist, nurses, and social workers should work together to pinpoint the individual characteristics of your cancer and to design a customized treatment regimen based on these diagnostic details.

Remember, your breast cancer is NOT your mother's, your friend's, or your neighbor's breast cancer. Individualized diagnosis is critical for every woman suspected of having this disease.

❖ What should I do if my various doctors disagree about how to treat my breast cancer, and they're giving me conflicting and confusing information?

The biggest surgical decision you will make is whether to save your breast (with the lumpectomy procedure) or to have your breast removed (with the mastectomy procedure). This choice should be based on the size and extent of your breast tumor, the size and shape of

Make them duel.

your breasts, and your personal feelings, among other factors. As I will discuss further in the treatment chapter, for women with small, early cancers, lumpectomy followed by radiation to the breast offers equal survival rates to complete removal of the breast. However, not all doctors present the choice in this manner. If two doctors give you differing recommendations on this subject, then a third tie-breaker opinion can be very valuable. (See page 129 for a discussion of how to go about finding second or third opinions). Always listen to the rationale of a specialist before making any major decisions, however. Why? Because specialists may be able to give you the latest information in their field, while your family doctor—though well-meaning and perhaps very intelligent—just can't keep up with every advance in all areas of medicine.

Of course, there are other issues doctors can squabble about, too—such as what type of incision should be made during surgery, what type of reconstruction to do after mastectomy, which chemotherapy regimen to choose, whether or not to take hormonal therapy after chemotherapy is done, and many other such issues. What are you to do about that? First, it's vital to find a doctor whose opinion you trust, and who you feel should act as captain of your team. This should be a physician you are interested in working with to maintain your health over a lifetime, not just during the acute phase of your breast

LIST OF QUESTIONS TO ASK YOUR DOCTOR:

1. Can a needle biopsy spread my breast cancer?

2. Is my cancer invasive or noninvasive?

3. What size is my tumor?

4. Is my tumor fast or slow growing?

5. Can you tell what stage my cancer is in? (Your doctor can only give you an idea at this point, before surgery is done.)

6. Do I have to have my lymph nodes removed?

7. Do you perform sentinel node biopsy, and what is your false negative/accuracy rate?

8. What are my surgical options for treatment?

1. Who was Erica Kane's third husband?

2. What are the ingredients in Chubby Hubby ice cream?

3. What is the square root of 6,763?

4. Who is your favorite Brady?

5. Do you know the way to San Jose?

9. Do I need radiation after surgery?

10. Do I need chemotherapy?

11. What will I feel like and look like after surgery?

12. Can I have breast reconstruction at the time of my surgery?

13. If I do not have reconstruction of my breasts at the time of surgery, can I use a prosthetic breast? How can I obtain one?

14. When will I be able to work after surgery?

15. How soon after my diagnosis will I need surgery?

16. What can I eat before surgery, and when should I stop eating?

17. Do I have to tell people at work about my diagnosis?

18. Will I have to stop taking hormones, and if so, what can I do about menopausal symptoms?

19. Can I work during radiation therapy or chemotherapy?

20. When can I resume my normal life activities again—such as sex and exercise?

Note: Your doctor may not be able to answer some questions completely until surgery is performed.

cancer treatment. When you have a key, trusted physician orchestrating your care, all decisions are made much more easily.

But you don't just want to drop the ball in your doctor's lap, either. It's important to take a crash course in breast cancer yourself, in order to familiarize yourself with the issues at hand. How can you do that during the stressful time of breast cancer diagnosis? For starters, bring a pad and pen, and ideally, another set of listening ears to your doctor visits. Having a companion at your side can help a great deal when you're trying to absorb an enormous amount of new information all at once. Later, when you get home, you can talk to your companion—a spouse, partner, parent, adult child, friend—and together sort out some of the more complicated issues. If you can't bring a companion with you, consider bringing a tape recorder so you can share the information with loved ones later on, or simply review the conversation yourself when you are feeling more calm. Above all else, ask every question that comes to your mind. Don't fear looking stupid in your doctor's eyes—you are not expected to be an expert. Far better to ask questions in the beginning and help to make smart choices about your care, than to remain mute and feel disappointed later.

◆ How else can I educate myself about breast cancer?

You've already started—by reading this book. And there are many other ways to educate yourself about breast cancer as well. For instance, the Internet is a good source of information, but beware of chat rooms, which can suffer from a lack of quality control. Many strong organizations now have information available online, including the National Cancer Institute, the American Cancer Society, the National Alliance of Breast Cancer Organizations, and the National Breast Cancer Coalition, among others. (See the Resources section, pages 265–296, for many additional on-line and other information sources.) Your doctor or hospital may have pamphlets filled with basic information about the disease (we do). In the back of this book, we have listed many different resources where you can call or write for detailed information on breast cancer and its treatment. The bottom line is this: The better educated you are about your condition, the greater your chance of making smart choices in face of the differing medical opinions that you may encounter as you go through the diagnostic and treatment process.

◆ I WANT A SECOND OPINION. HOW SHOULD I PLAN FOR IT, AND WHAT ABOUT THE SENSITIVE ISSUE OF MY OWN DOCTOR'S FEELINGS?

Forget about your doctor's feelings; this is a time to worry about yourself. You are making major decisions about your future life and health. Hopefully, your doctor has your best interests at heart and is giving you the best information and advice he or she has. But you are en-

Practice saying it in front of a mirror: "I want a second opinion."

titled to hear another point of view. So if you don't feel comfortable with your doctor's recommendations, feel a need for more information, or simply want to hear another medical authority echo your own doctor's words, by all means seek a second opinion.

There are, however, several key things to keep in mind when going for your second opinion visit. First, you must arrive prepared. Bring your current mammogram and any other imaging tests that have been done to diagnose your condition. Ideally, also bring originals of your last one or two mammograms from years past—these will help the doctor assess the significance of any apparent change. Copies just don't have the same clarity. Also be sure to bring your pathology report and any other written reports you have received from your original doctor(s), as well as your actual pathology slides. These are glass slides, which are usually placed in plastic containers or in cardboard mailers. If you find yourself sitting in your doctor's office but forgot to bring your pathology slides, you can fax a release form to the pathology department and ask that the slides be sent directly to your doctor. The release form must be signed by you, not by your doctor. By the way, all of these written and physical materials are rightly yours and should be safeguarded for possible future use. Finally, ask your pathology department to save your tissue in the event that it might be useful down the road. For instance, it may someday be possible to run new tests on your old tissue, tests that could reveal valuable information in light of new breast cancer treatments. Store your original mammograms in a safe place or return them to the mammogram facility. And keep copies of all paperwork related to your case in a file.

◆ HOW CAN I CHOOSE A DOCTOR FOR MY SECOND OPINION?

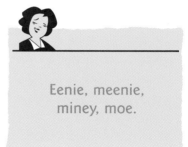

Eenie, meenie, miney, moe.

I certainly understand that it might be awkward to ask your own doctor for a recommendation—and in any case, you probably want someone from outside your doctor's "orbit." I recommend several approaches. First, talk to friends or family members who were happy with their breast cancer treatment. Sometimes a personal recommendation is the best of all. Also, call your family doctor or primary health care provider and ask for names of colleagues who specialize in breast cancer treatment. If you particularly like your hospital or another reputable one nearby, ask if it offers a second opinion referral service.

Now, a few words about the results of your second opinion visit. If the second doctor agrees with your own physician, you may now be comfortable moving forward with a given treatment regimen. If, on the other hand, the doctors disagree in some substantive way, ask them to communicate with each other—in your presence. A telephone conference call, for example, would allow you to hear the doctors converse and defend their own views. This could help you to choose a side, or, in some cases, to seek a third "tie-breaker" opinion. Now, I've seen women who get so confused and caught up in the cycle of opinions that they see four, five, six, or more doctors, delaying needed treatment before making important decisions. This certainly should not be your goal. But there is nothing wrong with doing a little digging to get to an answer with which you are at least intellectually comfortable—even if you are still emotionally scared.

A final possibility to keep in mind is that your case really may be slightly unusual or tricky, leaving room for doctors to view it different ways. If this is true, you might ask your doctors if they would be willing to present your case at a meeting known as a "breast conference"—where a consensus of opinion can be reached among a larger number of breast care specialists. Patients often don't know that such a conference exists. But these days, not only major teaching hospitals but also many community hospitals offer this helpful service. It's certainly worth asking if such an option might be available in your case.

◆ I JUST READ A COPY OF MY BREAST CANCER REPORT AND IT LOOKS LIKE A FOREIGN LANGUAGE. HOW CAN I READ AND UNDERSTAND IT?

Read your report with your doctor, and ask that every single item be fully explained. Anything confusing should be translated into plain English. Sometimes, for instance, it's not a simple matter of benign or malignant—that is, harmless or cancerous. There are certain condi-

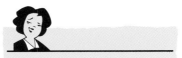

Perdon, no entiendo la pregunta.

tions which are deemed "benign" on a lab report that are, in fact, indicative of increased risk. Such conditions require varying degrees of follow-up with your doctor. Make sure it is absolutely clear whether you need to be examined in any special way, or at any unusual intervals, to check for changes in your

◆ ◆

condition. This is no time to be shy. Ask any and all questions right up front.

◆ ARE THERE BETTER AND WORSE TYPES OF BREAST CANCER DIAGNOSES?

Yes. Breast cancers are characterized in several ways, to help doctors determine how aggressive they are, how advanced, and so on. Three key factors we look at include (1) the size of the tumor, (2) whether the cancer has spread to the lymph nodes, and (3) whether the cancer has spread to other parts of the body (known as metastatic disease). In general, bigger tumors are worse than smaller ones; cancers that have spread to the lymph nodes are more worrisome than those that have not; and cancers that have metastasized to other parts of the body are of greater concern than those that have not yet spread. This does not mean, however, that larger cancers that have spread beyond the breast are impossible to treat. On the contrary, we are successfully treating all types and degrees of breast cancer these days.

Tests are done to determine the various important characteristics of the breast cancer cells, and these tests may be used to guide treatment decisions. The most important pieces of information are the lymph node status (that is, whether the cancer has spread to these nodes); the size of the tumor; and a variety of important characteristics of the cancer cells—known as pathology findings. For instance, we will find out whether the cells are dividing fast—meaning that they are relatively aggressive; and we will look to see if the cells in the tumor are more uniform (better) or more bizarre-looking. There are many scientific terms for the characteristics we study—such as the "nuclear grade" of the cell (low, moderate, or high), the so-called histologic grade (what the whole tumor looks like), the "growth fraction," and many other off-putting terms. To help you navigate this new and foreign language of breast cancer, I have created the following chart to show which characteristics are indicative of less worrisome tumors, and which are of greater concern. Take your lab report and match the terms to the chart below:

PATHOLOGY TERMS AND GOOD/BAD RATINGS		
FACTOR	LESS WORRISOME LESS AGGRESSIVE	MORE WORRISOME MORE AGGRESSIVE
axillary lymph node status	negative nodes	positive nodes
histologic tumor type	tubular, papillary, medullary, colloid (or mucinous)	all others
tumor size	smaller (under 1.5 cm)	larger (over 1.5 cm)
nuclear grade	low	high
histologic grade	well differentiated	poorly differentiated
estrogen/progesterone protein receptors	positive	negative
DNA content	diploid	aneuploid
S-phase	less than 5 percent	greater than 5 percent
HER-2/neu	absent	present
p53	absent	present

Finally, keep this in mind: If needed tests are not performed on your breast tissue the first time around, all is not lost—your slides can be taken out once again and the tissue retested. I frequently see patients who come from other hospitals without these needed tests. We simply take the tissue saved from the previous biopsy and start the pathology testing over from scratch.

And remember that all of these findings are your own, personal information and you are entitled to know about these details of your diagnosis. Such details not only help explain your prognosis, but also help to guide the treatment program you will eventually select. Always bear in mind that customization is the key to good breast cancer care. So the more detailed and personalized your diagnosis, the better tailored your treatment plan can be.

◆ HOW LONG DOES IT TAKE TO GET BIOPSY RESULTS?

All cells are processed in what's known as a "permanent section," which yields results in 24 to 48 hours and is extremely accurate. Far less often, cells are first processed in a so-called frozen section (in which the cells are immediately frozen in

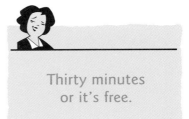

Thirty minutes
or it's free.

liquid nitrogen). The frozen section takes just a few minutes and yields 98–99 percent accurate results. I will do frozen sections only when I believe that immediate treatment decisions could change based on the results. One caveat everyone's doctor should bear in mind is that the frozen section should not be used when operating on calcium. This is because during the freezing process, calcium can fall off and the tiny area of concern may not be identified. You might want to ask your doctor about his or her policy on this matter.

◆ SHOULD I BREAK THE NEWS ABOUT MY CANCER DIAGNOSIS TO MY CHILDREN?

I'd like to let two of my patients answer this question. Their experience in dealing with their children holds important lessons for all women. The bottom line is both you, and the children, can benefit tremendously from the right kind of openness:

Laura (children aged nine and eleven at the time of her diagnosis): I found out in the evening. It was a situation in which I was sure the biopsy was normal, not cancer. When the doctor called in the evening and said it was malignant, nine months after my husband died of cancer, it was really quite a shock. I wasn't at that time prepared to tell the kids. But by the end of the evening, the kids knew something was up. They're perceptive. The school psychologist said not to tell the kids right away. But by morning, I felt I should tell them, and after further conversations, the school psychologist agreed with me. Better to tell them, better to be honest. Honesty is much better. I learned this through their father's illness. I decided to be as straightforward as I could. My son's initial reaction was incredible anger, since his father lived only three weeks after he was diagnosed with cancer. He said, "You're going to be dead by New Year's." I knew that I would not die like his father had. But all I could do to prove that to him was to stay alive.

Later, I had to have another biopsy. Some people don't tell their kids about biopsies because they don't want them to experience the pain of it. But I thought it would be better to tell them so that if something was found, they would be prepared. If nothing was found, they would learn that not all news is bad news. The second biopsy was normal, thank God.

They still tell me about things, when they're having a hard time dealing with their father's death or their fears about something happening to me. I have gotten lots of letters from people after my husband died, telling me that when their parent died, no one told them about it, so everyone else mourned together and then, when they learned much later what happened, they felt very much alone. I think my kids are much more open about talking to me about things, partly because I was open with them. My daughter talks about things I wouldn't talk about with my parents—her period, boys, and so on.

There is a line beyond which you don't tell your kids things—your own fears, for example. Finding that line is important. You need to protect them, but not shelter them.

Susan (adult children when diagnosed): When I was first diagnosed, I called my oldest son right away. He was thirty-seven. He came over with a big flowering plant. The important thing is to not keep it a secret. The reality when you first hear the news is horrible—a horrible reality. It helps a lot to share it with people that you love, people that are close to you. It's very important at first, when you first hear the news. I also have two other sons. The two that live near me came to the hospital for the whole day during my surgery, and they were there again during a second surgery. I found it very, very supportive to be surrounded by love. They became part of it. I met the doctor with my sons present. They waited in the waiting room and then asked the doctor questions of their own afterward. You have to make your family and friends part of this. Once before, I was sick and didn't tell them about it and they were very upset later.

I HAVE BEEN DIAGNOSED WITH BREAST CANCER. WHAT OTHER TESTS SHOULD I HAVE TO DETERMINE IF THE CANCER HAS SPREAD ELSEWHERE IN MY BODY?

If the cancer was found on a physical exam by your health care provider, but not yet visualized on a mammogram, you should have a mammogram to check the rest of your breast, and your other breast, for any additional abnormalities. You should also

◆ ◆

have a chest X ray to determine the unlikely event that the cancer has invaded your lungs, and a variety of blood tests to look for any abnormalities that could signal that the cancer has spread to other vital organs. These same tests may also be required by the anesthesiologist before you can be given any anesthesia. A blood test that reveals abnormal liver function could lead to further testing, such as a CAT scan.

If your breast cancer was caught early, chances are you will not be given an extensive workup to look for cancer spread. For instance, I do bone scans and CAT scans on women with extensive breast cancer, but not among women with tiny, node-negative breast cancer, as there is an exceedingly low chance of finding any abnormalities in this latter group. On the other hand, if a woman absolutely wants more extensive testing for peace of mind, I will certainly order it, even though it is not cost-effective (i.e., the cost of the test doesn't warrant the minute chance of finding something abnormal). The fact is, there are good and bad reasons to do bone scans. On the downside, a bone scan can lead to ambiguous findings, which lead to further testing and further anxiety. For instance, arthritic changes in the bones can raise a flag on the bone scan, leading to still further investigations that will likely yield no problem at all. On the plus side, a clear baseline bone scan can be used as a guide when reading bone scans in later years—if there's no change, there's no worry. So you can see an argument can be made both for doing and for not doing the scan. All factors taken into consideration, I personally have moved away from doing these scans in women with the earliest cancers.

Furthermore, if I find that the breast cancer is more extensive than we originally thought—let's say, for instance, that there are more lymph nodes involved—a more extensive workup including CAT scans of the chest and abdomen will be performed later. So you see, just as the diagnosis and treatment of breast cancer must be tailored to the individual woman's case, so the overall cancer workup should be customized to meet the needs of each and every woman.

DIAGNOSIS

A	G	V	H	G	M	T	E	M	V	O	E	W	K	W	Y
X	V	N	T	H	Z	G	Y	E	W	X	Q	D	Y	D	S
W	R	Q	O	H	X	Q	H	I	E	U	S	D	R	E	P
Z	J	Y	V	G	A	N	X	I	E	T	Y	U	U	L	D
I	S	E	D	O	N	H	P	M	Y	L	V	P	N	D	R
R	I	O	O	W	P	I	I	J	M	M	T	E	M	N	S
A	G	X	S	P	B	U	G	A	S	F	B	C	M	P	L
B	S	C	T	X	N	P	M	A	J	E	V	G	M	C	Q
R	F	B	K	N	I	O	S	E	T	Z	N	U	O	Y	J
I	M	A	R	G	O	M	M	A	M	S	L	U	C	S	P
L	V	Z	B	S	N	K	N	F	C	G	C	C	O	T	T
M	N	O	I	T	A	C	I	F	I	C	L	A	C	O	Y
I	C	Y	T	U	M	O	R	Q	Q	Z	U	I	T	Q	F
Z	L	U	Z	D	O	B	I	O	P	S	Y	P	C	Q	V
B	S	R	Y	B	O	M	A	S	S	D	C	P	F	R	S
C	V	I	Q	O	W	P	S	A	N	G	E	R	O	P	B

Find and circle the following words:

ANGER	CYST	MASS
ANXIETY	LUMP	STAGING
BIOPSY	LYMPH NODES	TUMOR
CALCIFICATION	MAMMOGRAM	

5

THE FIGHT:
Breast Cancer Treatment

JILL EIKENBERRY

I'll never forget the day I was diagnosed. I went to the breast specialist, and he told me I had breast cancer. I was devastated. I had thought he would have to do surgery or something to find out for certain, but he knew immediately that it was malignant, he could tell from the mammogram. I was very sure I was going to die. I hadn't ever really known anybody who had breast cancer—the only woman I knew who had it was the woman who lived upstairs from my apartment in New York, who had died the year before, leaving three children behind. That was my experience with it. And so I really thought it was a death sentence. It was really hard to hear what the doctor had to say after the words "breast cancer." I couldn't really be present. I was going to die.

After explaining the difference between mastectomies and lumpectomies, my doctor recommended a mastectomy because he was a conservative doctor and that's what he did most frequently. And I said sure, take it off. Whatever you have to do. Get it off me. So my husband and I went home in despair. We thought it was the end. I remember I had this long, dark hallway in my apartment in New York and as I was walking up and down that hallway, I thought, "You know, there's no light at the end of this tunnel." I really thought it was the end.

About three days after my diagnosis, I forced myself out of bed, got dressed, and went to a screening of a movie that I had done with John Lithgow called The Manhattan Project. *I wasn't going to tell anybody about this horrible thing, because I had just done the pilot for L.A. Law, I was about to start the whole series, and I didn't want to be known as "The Woman With Cancer." And so I walked into the lobby of the movie theater, and ran into Cynthia Nixon, a young actress who was also in the movie. She took one look at my face and said, "What happened?" And I just started pouring out the whole story to her right there in the lobby.*

She took me into the audience where her mom was sitting, and her mother took me by the hand, dragged me into the ladies' room, hiked up her blouse, and showed me this little scar on her right breast, and said, "See that? That's all I have left to remind me of my breast cancer eleven years ago." Right there, in the ladies' room, it occurred to me for the first time that I might not die from this disease. That was the moment I got the courage to seek a second opinion. And the second doctor told me that I was a perfect candidate for a lumpectomy. So I ended up saving my breast because this woman had the courage to show me her scar. A total stranger had the courage to show me her scar.

I KEEP HEARING ABOUT THE "BIG THREE" TREATMENTS FOR BREAST CANCER—WHAT ARE THEY AND WHEN DO YOU USE THEM?

The so-called big three treatments for breast cancer are (1) surgery, (2) radiation therapy, and (3) chemotherapy (which is a fancy name for medications used to fight cancer). I'll tell you a bit about each one and when it is used. Let's start with surgery, my own specialty.

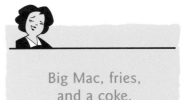

Big Mac, fries, and a coke.

BREAST CANCER SURGERY

Surgery involves an operation in which cancerous cells are literally cut out of the body. A variety of operations can be done, and they differ in terms of how much of the breast is taken away. For example, in the old days, surgeons often did a procedure called a "radical mastectomy," in which they removed not only the entire breast but the underlying chest wall muscle as well. This was a very disfiguring procedure, which we now know is not necessary to improve survival. Today, there are two equally effective options: in one, the modified radical mastectomy, the entire breast is removed (but not the underlying muscle); and in

Mastectomy Bikini

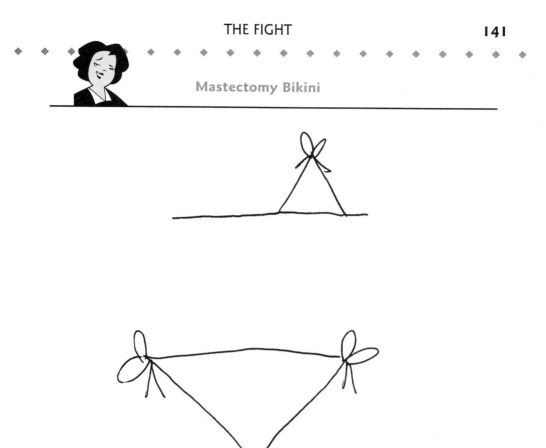

the other, called the lumpectomy procedure, just the cancerous lump is removed along with a rim of normal breast tissue from around the lump. The latest approach to mastectomy is called "skin-sparing" mastectomy. As its name suggests, this procedure involves the removal of the breast tissue, nipple, areola, and biopsy site—but leaves most of the breast skin intact. This skin preservation creates a better cosmetic result and also provides the skin laxity, which makes breast reconstruction easier. The lumpectomy procedure is usually followed by radiation therapy, which I'll discuss more in a moment. Other surgical procedures can be done that make up a middle ground between removing the entire breast and removing just the lump, such as a "quadrantectomy," which refers to removing one quadrant—or one-quarter—of the breast. It is rarely necessary to perform a quadrantectomy, however.

❖ How should I decide which surgical procedure is for me?

First, it's vital to debunk an old myth. Many women, and some doctors, still cling to the old belief that more is better—that is, taking more of the breast away will increase your chance of survival. This simply is not true. Studies have shown that

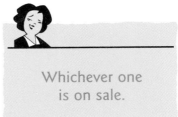

Whichever one
is on sale.

the lumpectomy procedure produces an equivalent survival rate to full removal of the breast. So the first thing to remember in making this big decision is that the breast-sparing choice is an equally safe one. I always remind women, furthermore, that while I cannot tape on a breast that has been removed, you can always go back for *more* surgery if for any reason the lumpectomy procedure is not successful. Most women never come back for more.

However, the lumpectomy procedure is not for everyone. There are several contraindications to lumpectomy—that is, reasons *not* to have it done:

REASONS NOT TO HAVE LUMPECTOMY:

1. If you have two cancers in separate areas of the breast;

2. If you have diffuse or spread-out microcalcifications in your breast, and your doctors cannot ascertain if they all are benign;

3. If, after repeated surgeries, the edge of the excision (or margins of the resection) reveal malignant or cancerous cells;

4. If you are pregnant (certainly in the first trimester, when radiation therapy should not be used);

5. If you have had previous radiation therapy to the chest or breast region for Hodgkin's disease or another cancer, and cannot have radiation again;

6. If your breast is small compared to the size of the cancerous tumor, so that removing the tumor would create a poor cosmetic result;

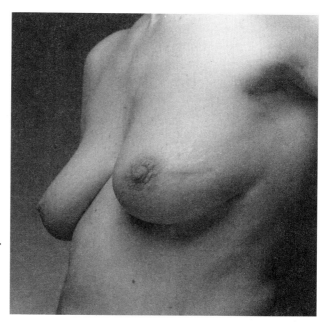

Lumpectomy scar

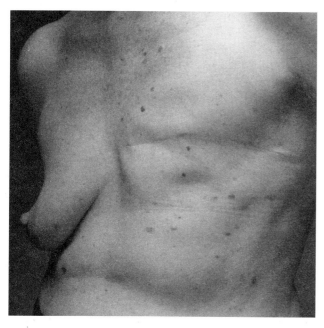

*Woman's chest
with mastectomy
and no
reconstruction*

7. If you have discharge from your nipple that is known to be cancerous, which suggests that the cancer might involve other parts of the breast;

8. If you have a connective-tissue disease, such as scleroderma, which can lead to a poor cosmetic result (and may or may not exacerbate the connective-tissue disease).

Also be attuned to recommendations that don't seem to jibe with what you know about the facts of your case. For example, if you have been told that you have a very small cancer, and your doctor is talking about doing a quadrantectomy (which removes more tissue than a lumpectomy does) or mastectomy, a bell should go off in your mind—this is too much surgery. It's like using a cannon to knock out a sand castle. Your goal should be to have the most appropriate conservative surgery possible for your particular case—or, if you *choose* a more extensive procedure, you should be making an educated, informed decision.

Three Women: Three Choices

Sharon (mastectomy with no reconstruction): There's something very "no muss, no fuss" about mastectomy without reconstruction. I have a prosthesis, we call her "boobsy." I'm a small-breasted woman, so it's easy for me. I wear shirts with pockets and fold a couple of tissues and get away with it—for me, it works very well. Reconstruction involved extra surgery, which I wasn't interested in. The surgery involved lots of time, or taking skin from another part of my body, and at the time it wasn't covered by insurance. The biggest adjustment for me was I had these really nice summer dresses that I couldn't wear with a bra, and I'm not into having my bra show so I can't wear them. But I feel fine the way I am right now; in fact, I don't use the prosthesis around the house. I'm married and my husband and I don't care about conventional appearances. Sometimes I wear it when I'm out if I don't want to look lopsided. I went to a woman dermatologist recently to have my skin checked, and she saw my prosthesis and said wow what a great prosthesis, it's beautiful, and she was admiring it and that helped a lot, made me feel good. I am how I am, and I feel fine about it.

May (mastectomy followed by reconstruction): I wasn't going to go ahead with reconstruction, but Dr. Axelrod spoke to me about it and looking back I'm glad I did. In my opinion, you get up in the morning and are confronted by your body. Without breasts, I knew I'd be reminded of the cancer. This way I'm not reminded of it constantly. At least there's something there. This makes you feel better. I look at myself and it doesn't bring back all those memories. I can forget about the cancer sometimes. I can look at myself and see a whole per-

REASONS WHY IT'S BETTER TO HAVE ONE BREAST:

1. When you're talking to a man, you know he'll be looking you in the eye at least half the time.

2. There's only a 50 percent chance of falling out of your bikini.

3. Half the sagging.

4. You could run for president, and your campaign slogan could be "Vote for Me, Because There are Already Enough Boobs in Government."

5. When parties get dull, you can whip out your prosthetic and play catch with it.

6. You can have your friends call you a tough-sounding nickname, like "Lefty."

7. No more awkward "purse-strap crossover."

son, not someone with a piece missing. When I look at my chest, I'm still a female, I have my breasts.

Pamela (lumpectomy): There were many variables when I was diagnosed. I hadn't been married or had kids. What do breasts mean to a young woman? I tried not to let this affect my decision about treatment. But I went deep down to my core, it sounds so hokey, but I asked myself what needs to be done here, is the cancer gone—and I felt that it really was gone. My doctor told me the margins around the tumor were clean. People ask how long are you a survivor, and for me, it's since the lump came out. I think psychologically there's a certain component looking down and seeing that you have the same body as before the surgery. I look down and my boobs are even, and I feel the surgery was so perfect. I have a new respect for my breast, I look down now and know that at one time I housed something that could have killed me. Now I meditate and get really quiet and know that inside my breast, it's now quiet in there, too.

◆ WHEN AND WHY ARE LYMPH NODES REMOVED?

Y our doctor may remove some of
your lymph nodes to see if the cancer has spread from your breast to
your body's lymph system. Lymph
nodes can be removed at the same
time as the surgery to remove your
cancerous lump or your breast.

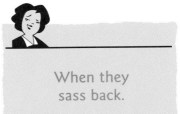

When they
sass back.

There are three different levels of lymph nodes that may be removed—the nodes closest to the "tail" of the breast (that is, the
upper outer portion), the nodes behind the small chest muscle,
and the nodes closest to the neck.

Although you might want to ask your doctor how many
nodes will be removed, it's impossible for your doctor to answer
this question before surgery, because different women have different numbers of lymph nodes. Heavier women tend to have more
than slimmer women, for example. Removing lymph nodes does
not improve your survival rate, but it does serve several important
roles: (1) it helps to determine the stage of your cancer, and

Location of Lymph Nodes

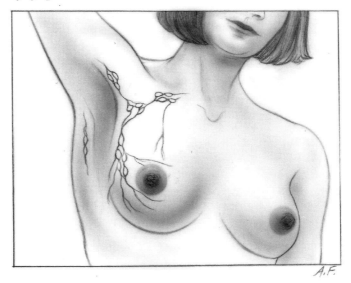

thereby give you an idea of your prognosis; (2) it helps guide the treatment process (along with lots of other information about the tumor, which you can find in the chart on page 133); and (3) it may help to locally control your disease in the armpit. Also, removing lymph nodes is helpful because many so-called clinical trials, in which women are given new anticancer treatments under formal scientific study, categorize women according to how many lymph nodes showed evidence of cancer. If your doctor doesn't take them out, there's no way to get this information.

◆ WHAT ARE THE RISKS OF BREAST CANCER SURGERY?

With all surgical procedures, there are potential risks and complications. These risks are minimized when you're in the hands of a competent surgeon. But they are never fully eliminated. The usual surgical risks include bleeding and infection.

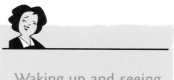

Waking up and seeing an ugly nurse.

With breast surgery, there is the additional risk of fluid collection in the breast (which, oddly enough, is actually a desirable "complication" in the case of lumpectomy, since it helps to shape the breast for a good final outcome). With mastectomy, however, you don't want fluid collection, because it creates a prolonged drainage problem for which tubes need to be left in place, or repeated aspirations are necessary to remove the fluid. And after lymph node dissections, prolonged fluid buildup also can lead to the need for repeat aspirations—which no one wants.

Other possible risks include nerve damage (rarely) and resultant numbness and discomfort. This can occur when the so-called intercostobrachial nerve (located in the underarm area) is removed or disrupted during breast surgery. *But this should rarely happen.* Talk to your doctor *before* you undergo surgery about protecting this underarm nerve. Another rare problem after breast cancer surgery is called a "winged scapula"—an unsightly protrusion of the shoulder blade associated with shoulder pain. Again, competent and careful surgeons create this kind of problem extremely rarely.

The most dreaded side effect of breast cancer surgery, however, is lymphedema—or major swelling in the arm after removal of the lymph nodes. I will discuss lymphedema in detail below.

◆ WHAT EXACTLY IS LYMPHEDEMA, AND CAN IT BE CURED?

Lymphedema is a problem that oc-curs in 15–25 percent of women after their lymph nodes have been re-moved. It involves a variable amount of swelling in the arm caused by the accumulation of lymphatic fluid that is not filtered back into the vessels in

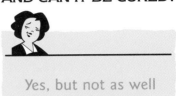

Yes, but not as well
as a ham.

the arm, and therefore escapes into the surrounding tissue. It may start out mild, and then insidiously develop into a serious disfigure-ment. Oddly enough, I have seen lymphedema set in shortly after lymph node removal, or as long as twenty years or more after the op-eration. The critical thing to remember is that whenever you see the first, minor sign of hand or arm swelling after lymph node removal, call your doctor. The faster you treat lymphedema, the better your chance of minimizing the terrible cycle of swelling, skin thickening, and fibrosis that can set in with time. See page 196 in the aftercare chapter for a complete discussion of how to manage lymphedema.

◆ HOW CAN I PREPARE FOR BREAST CANCER SURGERY?

A few major things to do before breast cancer surgery include:

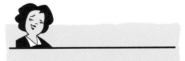

Ring Dings, and Ring
Dings only.

• Avoid drugs and vitamins that promote bleeding, such as aspirin, nonsteroidal anti-inflammatory drugs (such as Motrin, Advil, and Na-prosyn), and vitamin E for about five to seven days before surgery.

• Don't eat or drink after midnight the night before surgery if general anesthesia or intravenous sedatives will be used.

• If you are feeling extremely anxious before surgery and know that you will be having a procedure with just local anesthesia (some biopsies, for example), ask your doctor for a sedative to help you calm down.

• To assuage your fears about postoperative pain, talk to your doctor about whether he or she prescribes painkillers or uses a long-acting local anesthetic. These can help fight pain long after the procedure is done, so that you can go home feeling relatively comfortable.

• If you are having a procedure that requires that your doctor see your mammography films again, be sure you have control of your mammograms or know exactly where they are at the time of surgery. I've seen women forget about this under the stress of surgery, and a search must be undertaken, which delays the operation.

• If you have young children and know that you will be in the hospital overnight—or even if you are going for outpatient surgery but know that your children are frightened about it— give an important personal item of yours to the children to hold for you until you get home. Good choices include keys, glasses, and other items that your children know you need every day. This will help your kids to have confidence that you're coming back soon.

Of course, there are dozens of other ways to prepare for breast cancer surgery, both psychologically and practically. Some are as simple as going out to the movies with a supportive friend or family member the night before, to relieve some stress. I also recommend bringing a cassette recorder with headphones to the operating room, so that you can listen to your favorite music during the preparation phase.

◆ What can I expect after breast cancer surgery?

That depends on what type of surgery you have, and how extensive it is. Here are a few scenarios:

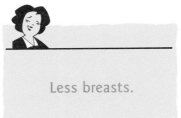

Less breasts.

A lumpectomy is an ambulatory procedure—that is, you will go home the day of your operation. This is good in some ways and not so good in others. On the plus side, many women want to be in the comfort of their own homes and to know that the procedure they have undergone is routine and uncomplicated. On the other hand, sometimes loved ones fail to recognize the seriousness of this treatment for breast cancer and don't give the kind of support and attention many women need afterward. They simply assume that if you can get home in a few hours, things must not be so dire. This is just one of countless reasons why it's so important to communicate with your closest support system, be that a spouse or partner, adult children, friends, or anyone else whose support you expect after surgery.

With the lumpectomy procedure, no drains should be used, so you don't have to deal with draining the breast when you get home, as many patients with more extensive breast surgery do (the cosmetic result can be pretty terrible when drains are used after lumpectomy, so talk to your doctor about this beforehand). When I have a patient who is really filled with fluid, I take out as much as I can, but not enough to create a defect— that is, I allow some of that extra fluid to help create a nice shape to the breast after the operation.

Patients may put a cold pack on the breast to reduce pain at home, but frankly, if a good long-acting local anesthetic is used during the operation, most women feel comfortable enough and don't need the cold pack. I also recommend that you buy a good, supportive sports bra for use after surgery— and even that you wear the bra to bed for a couple of nights after surgery. The compression offered by the bra helps stabilize the breast after surgery, which really helps speed recovery.

If more extensive surgery is done, there are more things to deal with after surgery. For example, if you have lymph nodes removed to see if cancer has spread there, you may have a drain in place which you will need to use for a maximum of about five days after surgery. (If a so-called sentinel node biopsy is done—a procedure I'll discuss in a moment—then a drain is not needed). I have finally found a great use for those fanny packs people wear around their waist instead of carrying a purse: the fanny pack can hold the drain bulb, which collects the fluid draining from the lymph system. It gives new meaning to "pack and go." Also, it's important to wear loose clothing after lymph node removal. Tunic-style attire is best, as it leaves the arms and armpits free and comfortable.

If you have a mastectomy—removal of the entire breast rather than just the cancerous lump—your postoperative experience will also be more involved. To begin with, you're likely to spend the night in the hospital. (It is now required by law that your insurance company and hospital allow you to stay overnight, as a reaction to the "drive-through" mastectomy mills that have gotten so much attention of late.) Truth be told, I have found that many women neither want nor need to stay overnight after a so-called total mastectomy, in which no lymph nodes are removed. The main need for assistance afterward is pain control and drainage, both of which can be handled at home. However, the modified radical mastectomy—in which the breast and lymph nodes are removed—requires more involved aftercare, and the vast majority of patients want and need a night in the hospital. With the modified radical mastectomy, two drains may be inserted—which is harder for the patient to manage. After one day, one of the drains is usually removed, making it easier to care for yourself. The nice thing to keep in mind is that only a decade ago, women were kept in the hospital for a week to ten days after mastectomy or lymph node surgery. Thanks to improved education, excellent outpatient nursing care, better pain control, and other factors, this procedure is much less psychologically and physically taxing than it used to be. I always tell my patients that it is perfectly normal if it takes their heads longer to recover from breast cancer surgery than it takes their bodies.

Finally, if you've had breast reconstruction following a mastectomy, your follow-up care and time in the hospital may differ. For example, if you have had an expander (a type of implant) put in, you might stay in the hospital for three days or so. If you have the belly-flap procedure discussed later on page 153, you may spend as long as a week in the hospital, and you should be given a pump so that you can self-administer intravenous pain medication as needed. Talk to your surgeon about what to expect with your particular case.

As for your diet and other behavior after breast cancer surgery, times have changed in this case as well. Doctors used to uniformly tell women to start with clear fluids and only gradually move up to a normal diet after breast cancer surgery. I think this is silly—in fact, I tell my patients that I didn't operate on their teeth or their stomachs—so if they want to eat a favorite food after surgery, by all means they should do it. Thanks to better anesthetics, fewer women are nauseated after surgery these days. On the flip side, while you *must* be well hydrated after surgery (fluids are important), you don't *have* to eat a steak if you don't want to. It is quite important to get up and move soon after surgery, to reduce the risk of such problems as blood clots and pneumonia. Again, I tell patients that I didn't operate on their legs—and that they can and should walk as soon as possible. The goal is to move as quickly as possible away from the notion of yourself as an invalid and into a vigorous, active life after surgery. Remember that breast cancer usually affects otherwise healthy women. After successful treatment for breast cancer, that otherwise healthy woman should thrive.

YOU'VE ALREADY HAD YOUR LEFT BREAST REMOVED . . . NOW HERE ARE SOME USES FOR THE LEFT CUP OF YOUR BRA:

1. A yarmulke with a chin strap

2. A planter

3. A dish for guest soap

4. A decorative ashtray

5. A knee pad

6. A lovely potpourri dish

◆ **I** KNOW THAT SOME WOMEN HAVE THEIR BREASTS RECONSTRUCTED AFTER CANCER SURGERY. HOW IS THIS DONE AND WHAT'S THE COSMETIC RESULT?

There are several ways to reconstruct the breasts after mastectomy, and these days a good plastic surgeon can do a remarkably natural-looking job. Ideally, reconstructive surgery is done immediately following breast cancer surgery—while the woman is still on the operating table—rather than making women go through another entire surgical experience at some time down the road. Often, the reconstructive procedure is chosen according to the woman's own body type. For instance, we like to use something called "autologous tissue flaps," with muscle, skin, and fat taken from the woman's own belly area. The procedure, which I tend to favor, is called the TRAM-flap procedure—for Trans Rectus Abdominus Musculocutaneous flap procedure. It can be done with or without additional complex and time-consuming microsurgery to reattach the blood vessels of the muscles you're grafting. Personally, I have had such success without the blood vessel surgery that I don't usually bother with it. However, some women—such as heavy smokers, or those with diabetes—may need the microvascular surgery to help provide extra blood flow to the flap.

But if a woman has little or no belly fat, or multiple abdominal surgical procedures with scarring (e.g., from cesarean sections or hysterectomy) the TRAM-flap procedure might not be possible. (If you do have excess belly fat, by the way, you can get the benefits of using it for your breast reconstruction—as well as the added benefit of an automatic "tummy tuck" built into the procedure!)

But there are other procedures as well. For instance, you can use tissue expanders to gradually loosen the skin of the chest and then use some type of artificial implant to create the look of a breast. Because of enormous recent controversy over their safety, silicone implants are now used only under scientific study in special cases, but saline (salt water–filled) implants are often used, and sometimes other types, such as soybean oil implants, are also used. Implants should be placed behind the chest muscles. They tend to be more secure when located there. But there are still problems with saline implants—including a less-natural-looking contour and feel than the older silicone implants. Sometimes rippling is visible. And they are more subject to rupture on impact, such as in an automobile accident.

In some procedures, muscles can be taken from the woman's back or from her buttocks for use in breast reconstruction. The bottom line is this: Do not settle for the first type of reconstruction you hear about. Ask for a good defense of why a particular form of reconstruction is being recommended for you, and what your surgeon's experience is in doing it. Ideally, choose a surgeon who does more than one type of procedure, so he or she will not be biased toward one particular approach.

But as they say, a picture tells a thousand words, and it's far better to look at pictures of actual reconstructed breasts than to imagine what they look like. Ask your doctor for pictures of his or her work, and also ask to be connected with another patient who might be willing to show her reconstructed breasts in person. This is common in my office.

See pages 156–157 for some examples.

Unfortunately, even with the great success of breast reconstruction in the hands of a talented surgeon, only a fraction of women have reconstruction done immediately after breast cancer surgery. I believe that this is because many women are still not given this important treatment option. So if your doctor doesn't raise the subject, be sure to bring it up yourself long before your breast cancer surgery is done.

◆ IS THERE ANYTHING I CAN'T DO AFTER BREAST RECONSTRUCTION?

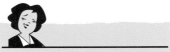

After the TRAM-flap reconstruction, for the first twenty-four hours after surgery, your bed will be adjusted to a certain angle to decrease the tension on the operation site. But quite soon you will be encouraged to get up and move. You will

You probably still won't be able to do that triple-lutz.

likely use special stockings on your legs to help prevent blood clots, and you'll have a catheter to remove urine from your bladder (the catheter will be taken out as soon as you start moving around). The day after surgery, you should be able to sit in a chair; and shortly thereafter you will gradually get up and walk around. You may be given a pain medicine pump so that you can control the amount and timing of your pain medication—but you can't count on this. Talk to your doctor about it ahead of time.

Some women remain hunched over for several days after surgery, while others walk upright immediately. Some go back to work in just a few weeks; others need as much as two months to get back to their normal selves. There may be a few permanent limitations on your mobility—though they are few

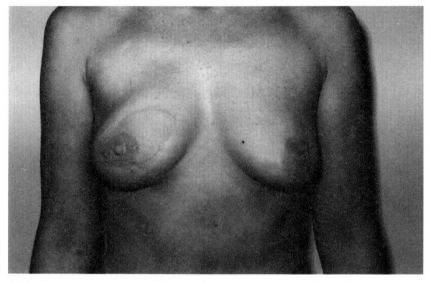

Right breast mastectomy and TRAM-flap reconstruction and nipple reconstruction

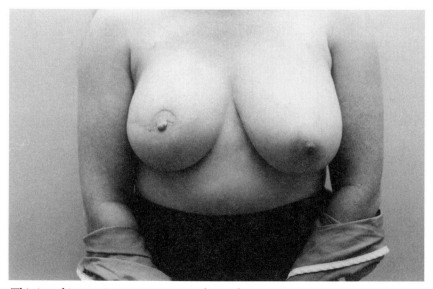

This is a skin-sparing mastectomy with nipple reconstruction

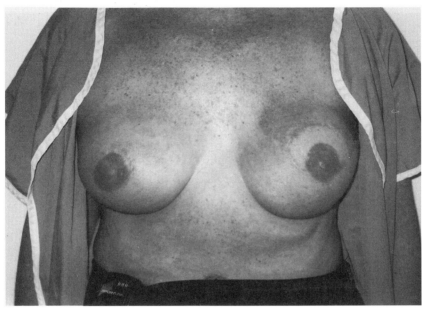

Bilateral mastectomy and TRAM-flap reconstruction with both nipples reconstructed

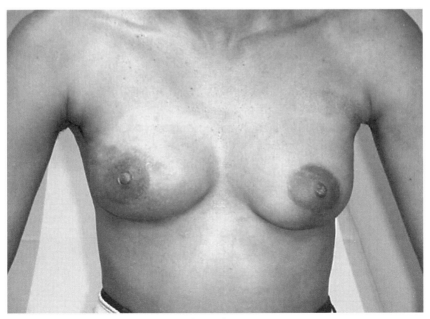

Right mastectomy with implant and nipple reconstruction

NOW THAT YOU'VE SURVIVED BREAST CANCER
AND HAD BOTH BREASTS REMOVED, LET'S GO OVER
WHAT YOU HAVE TO LOOK FORWARD TO
WITHOUT BREASTS:

1. No more embarrassing hard nipples when the wind blows.

2. No more wondering about the Wonderbra.

3. No more tossing and turning in pain when it's that time of the month.

4. No more bouncing when running downstairs.

and minor. For example, it might be hard to do a complete sit-up exercise—though not impossible. And you may not be a champion rower after breast reconstruction, as a result of some limit in your range of motion. But generally, you should come to feel just fine and to resume a vigorous regimen of physical activity and normal life tasks.

As for health problems after reconstruction, there are a few issues to consider. First, if implants are used, there is a chance of a problem called "capsular contracture," in which the implants and the tissue surrounding them contract and harden, creating discomfort and an abnormal appearance. If this occurs, the implant must be removed and a new one put in its place. Another potential problem is that implants can migrate from their proper place on the chest (this is less likely, though still possible, particularly when the implant is placed in front of the chest muscle rather than behind it). And of course, there is the risk of rupture—in which case the implant may appear smaller and will have to be removed. In addition, all of the standard risks of major surgery would apply here as well—including the small but real risks of infection and bleeding. If in the TRAM-flap procedure both stomach muscles were included in the reconstruction procedure, a graft may need to be put in to prevent hernias—but still, there may be a higher rate of hernias.

Finally, something that is just beginning to get more attention in the medical literature—but that is largely unknown to the general public—is the issue of so-called phantom breast pain after mastectomy with or without reconstruction. Women report feelings both of pain and of erotic sensations in the missing breast. This is not unlike the phantom limb sensations that arm or leg amputees talk about. The discomfort can be severe, but tends to lessen with time.

◆ IS THE NIPPLE RECONSTRUCTED TOO?

Yes, it can be, though not all women opt to have it done. In the past, we reconstructed nipples using skin from inside the inner thigh, since it was slightly darker than other skin and created a reasonable cosmetic result. Today, it is best done with tattooing, and with the wide range of color choices now available, the process of nipple reconstruction is not terribly unlike interior (or exterior) decorating of your own body! Women "shop" for the right color—with names such as "dusty rose," "sandstone," and "topaz." This is one part of the treatment process that actually brings a little levity to an otherwise serious situation.

Unfortunately, the reconstructed nipple does not have the sensation of a real nipple. But the appearance can be quite natural.

◆ WHAT IS RADIATION THERAPY?

Radiation therapy is similar to surgery in that it attacks breast cancer "locally"—i.e., inside the breast. Highly targeted, controlled radiation beams are directed at the breast tissue to kill off any cancer cells that may remain there after the cancerous tumor was removed. This is known as "sterilizing" the breast area—or, as I like to put it, it gives an extra "umph" in the fight to decrease the chance of breast cancer recurring inside the breast itself. Radiation is delivered daily in small amounts over a six- to seven-week period. Excessive amounts of radiation have the potential to kill normal healthy cells. When used in moderate, targeted doses, however, the healthy breast tissue is spared and the cancerous tissue is killed off.

If you have lumpectomy without radiation for invasive cancer, the chance of recurrence in the breast can be as high as 40 percent. Radiation cuts that number dramatically. Now remember—radiation treatment does not mean your overall survival is increased. But by reducing local recurrence rate (that is, the chance of the cancer coming back inside the breast itself), radiation therapy could save you unnecessary surgical procedures in the future. I should add, by the way, that there is a group of scientists and clinicians who believe that down the road we will prove that radiation therapy does indeed increase overall survival rates. But the data just aren't in yet.

The way radiation therapy is done today, there is little "scatter"—meaning that there is negligible damage to surrounding breast tissue or to the opposite breast, the esophagus, the heart, the lungs, and elsewhere. In the old days, women more often had burns on the skin, trouble swallowing, and other problems after radiation therapy. These days, those side effects are rare. You might get a little tanning of the breast skin and a little hardening or thickening of the breast, which significantly improves or even disappears over the next year. Sometimes there is swelling around the nipple and areola of the breast, but again, this is most often temporary. Some women find that their skin becomes extremely sensitive during radiation therapy. I recommend wearing light cotton clothing and using a variety of salves, like pure aloe gel, vitamin A and D ointment, and others, to maintain the integrity of the skin. Finally, some women feel tired when undergoing radiation therapy, which may be partly caused by the procedure itself and partly the result of dragging oneself back and forth between treatments and work (since many women go early in the morning, or late in the evening, to avoid disrupting their busy lives).

◆ ARE THERE SIDE EFFECTS TO RADIATION THERAPY?

On the plus side, there are no *obvious* side effects to radiation therapy—no hair loss, no nausea or vomiting, and other problems more commonly associated with certain kinds of chemotherapy for breast cancer.

> Your friends may say you're glowing.

One important thing to keep in mind before starting radiation therapy is that you can't start your treatment in one place and then continue it in another. You also can't take a break in the middle of radiation treatment. There is usually a two- to four-week break between breast surgery and the commencement of radiation therapy or chemotherapy, so if you want to take a needed vacation, this is a good time to do it. Many of my patients find that a vacation is a good way to unwind and to take a deep breath after the stress of surgery and before the beginning of more cancer treatments.

◆ IF MY CANCER HAS NOT SPREAD, WILL RADIATION BE USED?

Radiation may be used to treat noninvasive duct cell breast cancers or ductal carcinoma-in-situ (DCIS) but is not indicated for lobular carcinoma-in-situ (LCIS) cancers.

◆ WHAT IS CHEMOTHERAPY, AND WHO GETS IT?

Chemotherapy is, quite simply, using medication to fight cancer. There are many drug therapies available, including different combinations of drugs, different doses, different treatment order, and different timing, but the basic idea is the same:

Drugs fight cancer "systemically," which means they attack stray cancer cells throughout the body as a whole. Cancer drugs are given in groups, because it is known that several drugs together offer better protection than single agents.

> It's actually Keno-therapy. And old ladies need it to smoke and win some money on Saturday nights.

Drug treatment for cancer is quite different from surgery and radiation, which treat breast cancer inside the breast itself. The most common names of breast cancer drugs include Cytoxan, methotrexate, Adriamycin, 5-FU, and taxanes. (Taxol, a taxane, also an important weapon in the fight against ovarian cancer, is derived from the Pacific yew tree and has gotten widespread attention of late as an important addition to older-line breast cancer drugs.) Herceptin is also making its way into the breast cancer drug arsenal. Now recommended by the U.S. Food and Drug Administration for its effectiveness in treatment of breast cancer that has spread to distant sites in the body, Herceptin may soon be recommended for its effect on early breast cancers in certain groups of women as well.

Contrary to what many people believe, radiation and chemotherapy are not interchangeable. Every week, at least once, a patient asks me why, if she had chemotherapy already, does she also need radiation. The answer is quite simple. The surgery and radiation that treated the breast do nothing to fight cancer cells that may be lurking elsewhere in the body— and we don't yet have a tool with which to locate these hiding cells. Cancer drugs take up this fight where surgery and radiation cannot reach. The drugs are sometimes given through the veins, but it is also possible to put a "port" in a larger vein so drugs can be given continuously without destroying the veins in the arms. Then they travel throughout the blood system, doing their work to fight cancer cells. Some "ports" allow blood samples to be drawn as well, to help patients needing multiple blood tests to avoid feeling like pincushions.

Many women naturally worry about the side effects of chemotherapy. It should offer some consolation that the side effects sometimes accompanying chemotherapy, including nausea, vomiting, fatigue, and hair loss, are occurring for a good reason: that is, the "poison" that is making you feel sick is also wreaking havoc on your enemy, the cancer cells. A more serious side effect that can occur more commonly in women over forty is ovarian failure—or premature menopause—replete with typical menopausal symptoms such as mood changes, vaginal dryness and discomfort, hot flashes, sleep problems, and so on. In younger women, an important risk is infertility which can result from this ovarian failure. See page 180 for further discussion of this risk and whom it may more likely affect.

The use of chemotherapy has changed significantly in recent years. Only a decade ago, chemotherapy was reserved for women with so-called positive lymph nodes—that is, lymph nodes with cancer present in them. Today, both younger and older women with "negative" (cancer-free) nodes are given chemotherapy as well, especially if the tumor is greater than 1 cm in size (the size of your pinky nail). Also, ten years ago we used to give only the hormonal drug tamoxifen to older women with positive lymph nodes and tumors that are sensitive to the hormone estrogen (known as "estrogen receptor–positive" tumors). Today, we may give chemotherapy *plus* tamoxifen to these women. We often recommend that women who have estrogen receptor–positive tumors take tamoxifen twice a day for five years after completing chemotherapy.

◆ WHEN SHOULD A "PORT" BE USED TO DELIVER CHEMOTHERAPY?

If your chemotherapy nurses or doctors believe that your veins are insufficient to support your particular regimen of chemotherapy, a port may be used. Why might your "venous access" be in-

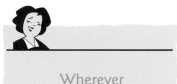

Wherever
there's a storm.

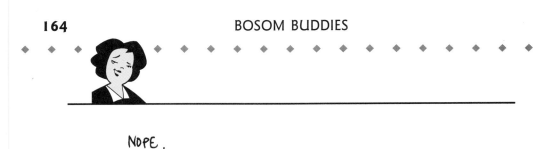

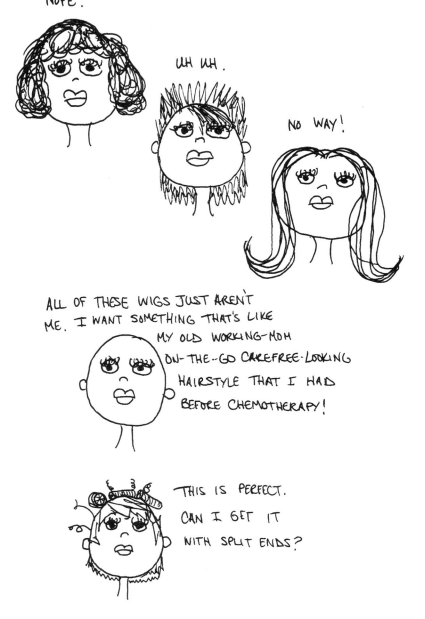

sufficient? Sometimes, when especially caustic chemotherapy drugs are used, small veins and your surrounding skin can suffer from burns and other skin irritation. Adriamycin is one example of a caustic chemotherapeutic drug commonly used to treat breast cancer.

Many women who have had lymph nodes removed during breast surgery are forced to receive chemotherapy in just one arm (the arm on the side of the body that did not have surgery). As a result, the veins in this one arm can be overused and may not suffice to get through chemotherapy. This is one case in which ports may be used.

Some women opt for a port from the get-go because it's easier and keeps the arms free of unpleasant pokes and bruises. And still other women start out with conventional treatment directly to the veins, but discover halfway through therapy that their veins cannot support the treatment, and switch to a port instead.

◆ WHY DO SOME PEOPLE HAVE CHEMOTHERAPY BEFORE SURGERY, AND OTHERS AFTERWARD?

The timing of chemotherapy, surgery, and radiation therapy has to do with a number of factors, such as the aggressiveness of the tumor. In general, it is more common for surgery to be done before chemotherapy. But there are a number of exceptions to this rule. For example, chemotherapy is given before other treatments in the case of a rare condition known as "inflammatory cancer," which is marked by redness and dimpling of the breast skin, usually without a palpable (feelable) mass. Another case in which chemotherapy is usually given before surgery is in the treatment of very large breast cancers. In this case, chemotherapy is given first in order to control disease outside the breast and to shrink the tumor as well—at which point it is possible, in some cases, to do a lumpectomy rather than a mastectomy. In this situation, doing chemotherapy before surgery may increase your survival rate. So you can see how critical it is for the various members of your cancer care team to communicate well *before* any treatments are started. Timing can be of the essence.

◆ ◆ ◆ ◆ ◆ ◆ ◆ ◆ ◆ ◆ ◆ ◆ ◆ ◆ ◆ ◆ ◆ ◆ ◆

◆ ARE THERE WAYS TO MINIMIZE THE SIDE EFFECTS OF CHEMOTHERAPY?

Yes. There are different ways to help reduce the various side effects of chemotherapy. For instance, there are medications that significantly reduce or prevent nausea and vomiting, such as the drugs Zofran, Kytril, or Compazine. Antinausea drugs (like Compazine and Norzine) can be taken at home soon after a chemotherapy session, before bothersome symptoms occur. If you wait until you're significantly nauseated and/or vomiting, the drugs are less helpful.

Most women with breast cancer have a passionate fear of hair loss, and it is not reassuring to them to hear that the hair will grow back (though it will). A lot of sexual and feminine identity is tangled up in that hair. While not all women will experience hair loss with chemotherapy, many will lose some if not all their hair during the treatment. The excellent

FIVE THINGS THAT MAKE YOU MORE NAUSEATED THAN CHEMOTHERAPY:

1. Peanut butter and mayo

2. How the sixty-seven-year-old leading man always hooks up with the twenty-one-year-old

3. Being forced to say: "The Artist Formerly Known as Prince"

4. Cheerleaders

5. The stuff on the string after you floss

anti–breast cancer drug Adriamycin is very likely to cause hair loss. Purchasing a natural wig that resembles your normal hair (or a stylish hat or turban) *before* hair loss sets in can help a great deal in keeping your self-esteem and self-image high at this difficult time. Although some recommend ice-cold packs on the head during chemotherapy to reduce the incidence of hair loss, the effectiveness of this treatment is controversial.

Another common side effect of chemotherapy is increased risk of infections, since the anticancer drugs impair the immune system partly by reducing the body's disease-fighting white blood cells. But we now have a very important drug called Neupogen, which boosts the number of white cells in the body and thereby reduces the risk of such infections.

Finally, a number of lifestyle changes can help make chemotherapy easier to bear. For example, eating numerous small meals throughout the day (including one small meal shortly before therapy) can help cut the risk of nausea. And doing whatever you can to make the chemotherapy process itself more tolerable is quite helpful to some women: for example, bring headphones with your favorite music to the treatment sessions. Some centers even offer relaxation techniques such as massage therapy in concert with chemotherapy treatments. Ask your doctor if you can be buddied up with a partner for chemotherapy—that is, another woman of similar age and condition who will be starting chemotherapy at the same time as you. Going through the treatment process together can lessen the fear and stress for both women. Also, if you work, ask for chemotherapy treatments on Friday so that you can recover over the weekend and be in good shape for Monday morning.

◆ IF I WANT TO HAVE CHILDREN AFTER CHEMOTHERAPY, SHOULD I HAVE MY EGGS HARVESTED AND FROZEN BEFORE I START CHEMOTHERAPY?

There are several issues to consider here. First, there is no standard technique for banking eggs. There are experimental techniques with high-dose ovarian hormone stimulation—which could be quite risky for a woman with breast cancer. It's

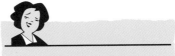

Yes, dye them pink and yellow.

more likely that you could consider banking *already fertilized* eggs—that is, embryos—for later implantation in your uterus. But this is a tricky matter as well, since hormonal stimulation is often (though not always) needed to make such pregnancies successful. Again, taking high-dose hormones for the first few months of pregnancy could be risky for a woman with a recent history of breast cancer. Certainly you should discuss this important issue with your own doctor and with a fertility specialist as well. Your type of tumor, stage of disease, age, and other factors will come into play when deciding whether this approach might be safe for you.

◆ ARE HORMONAL DRUGS PART OF CHEMOTHERAPY AND WHO GETS THESE TREATMENTS?

As far back as the 1890s, researchers learned that hormones play an important role in breast and other cancers. One important finding came about when women who lost their ovarian function early in life (under age thirty), and therefore stopped producing the hormone estrogen, had a dramatic reduction in their risk of breast cancer. We know today that many breast cancers are fueled by the hormone estrogen. Hormonal therapy is generally considered separate from chemotherapy, even though it too involves drug treatments to fight cancer. Hormonal therapy refers to the so-called designer estrogens, a group of drugs that have both *anti*-estrogenic and

THE ADVANTAGES OF CHEMOTHERAPY:

1. You don't have to pluck your eyebrows.

2. If you go to the Grammys, everyone will think you're Sinéad O'Connor.

3. You can use your Epilady to trim your hedge.

4. You don't have to worry about your bikini line when you visit your gynecologist.

5. When you break dance, it's easier to spin on your head.

6. No dandruff, no lice, no bad hair days.

7. No pigtails to be dipped in the ink well by that annoying person behind you at school.

estrogenic effects. They go by names such as tamoxifen, raloxifene, toremifene, droloxifene, and others—for which reason they are sometimes called the "fenes." Tamoxifen reduces the risk of recurrence and death from breast cancer. It's usually used after treatment for early breast cancer, but is also used for women with cancer that has spread to distant sites in the body. Another impressive finding is that tamoxifen cuts in *half* the risk of a second cancer developing in a woman's other breast. Tamoxifen is the only "fene" approved by the FDA for use in the treatment of breast cancer.

Formally, tamoxifen and its cousin drugs are known as SERMS—for selective estrogen receptor modulators. Tamoxifen is the most established of the SERMS, as it has been around since 1978. They are generally given to both older and younger women whose breast cancers are fueled by the hormone estrogen (so-called estrogen receptor–positive tumors). The drugs work by binding to the receptors on the tumor cells and thereby fooling the cell into thinking that it's being "fed" estrogen. With the receptor site covered, other estrogen in the body can't feed the cell. A variety of other processes are set off as well, many of which we don't fully understand as yet.

The so-called designer estrogens, which you can think of as fancier SERMS, are a group of drugs used in postmenopausal women because they seem to do the work of "good" estrogen but not the work of "bad" estrogen. On the plus side, they seem to help promote bone density and thereby fight osteoporosis; and they help promote a better blood cholesterol profile, reducing the risk of heart disease. They deter breast cancers, but they do *not* promote uterine cancer, as other forms of estrogen do. They represent an important medical breakthrough in that doctors have harnessed the best side effects of estrogen without the worst of it. Major studies are now under way to compare different members of the SERM family to see which ones are most effective against breast cancer, with the fewest side effects. For now, tamoxifen remains the gold standard against which these other drugs will be measured.

◆ WHAT ARE THE RISKS AND SIDE EFFECTS OF THESE HORMONAL DRUGS?

They are generally well tolerated, but about 5 percent of women will stop taking these drugs because of side effects. The side effects of tamoxifen are weight gain and a variety of menopausal symptoms, such as hot flashes, vaginal dryness, vaginal discharge, irregular menstrual

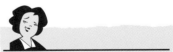

You may have a sudden desire to watch nonstop episodes of *The Love Boat.*

periods, and so on. The risks, though quite rare, include benign growth of the lining of the uterus, including polyps; ovarian cysts; uterine cancer; and thrombosis (life-threatening blood clots that can travel to the lungs). Rarely, it can worsen pre-existing cataracts and cause retinal problems in the eye. I recommend that women taking tamoxifen get regular gynecological exams and consult with their gynecologist as to which, if any, special test they should take. Aside from this, they must be sure to have their eyes checked regularly. Some doctors also recommend periodic endometrial biopsies—that is, tests of the lining of the uterus. Other members of the "fene" family of drugs are thought to have fewer side effects, but longer-term head-to-head comparison studies are needed to sort out such details.

◆ WITH SO MANY TREATMENT OPTIONS, HOW CAN I BE SURE WHICH TREATMENT IS RIGHT FOR ME?

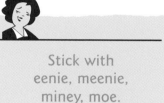

Stick with eenie, meenie, miney, moe.

The best treatment plan for breast cancer is the one that is customized to the particular kind of cancer you have. Customization comes about after a detailed diagnosis is made for your cancer. In the diagnosis chapter, we talk about a number of features of the tumor that affect treatment decisions. But another important thing to keep in mind is that there are two main types of breast cancer—"in-situ" breast cancer, and "invasive" or "infiltrating" cancer." Depending on which of these two main types of cancer you have, treatment will differ significantly.

◆ WHAT'S THE DIFFERENCE BETWEEN IN-SITU AND INVASIVE CANCER?

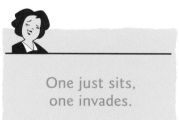

One just sits, one invades.

In-situ breast cancer refers to cancer that has not spread beyond the bottom part of the breast cell (called the "basement membrane")—that is, the tumor has not spread to anything surrounding the breast duct, for example, where it is located. Its name is the Latin words for "in place." Invasive or infiltrating cancers, on the other hand, have made their way out of their original location, and are therefore treated differently. Invasive cancer may or may not have spread out of the breast. Sometimes, the term just refers to cancers that have spread elsewhere in the breast, away from the original tumor site. Approximately 175,000 invasive breast cancer cases will be diagnosed this year in the U.S., and an additional 39,900 will be in-situ (noninvasive) cancer. The noninvasive cancers are caught early thanks to widespread screening mammography, the lifesaving breast X-ray tool discussed in chapter 2.

SO WHAT'S THE BEST TREATMENT APPROACH FOR NONINVASIVE BREAST CANCERS?

There are two main types of noninvasive or in-situ breast cancers. One, known as DCIS (for ductal carcinoma-in-situ), is an actual cancer which is located inside one of the breast ducts.

Sometimes these cancers are "well behaved" and not very aggressive; sometimes they are quite aggressive and will progress into a much more serious condition if left alone. DCIS is considered "stage 0" cancer—the earliest cancer you can catch. And in most cases, the breast can be saved. There are different types of DCIS, and I like to give my patients reading material to learn about the different forms. But in general, this is a relatively good type of breast cancer diagnosis. In fact, in the early 1980s, when widespread mammography screening was not yet routine, only 3 percent of cancers detected were DCIS; today, 30–40 percent of all breast cancers picked up by mammography are noninvasive or in-situ. This represents a major triumph in the detection of early, curable breast cancers.

The usual treatment for DCIS—lumpectomy plus radiation treatment—is equivalent in overall survival rates to the old gold standard treatment, mastectomy (removal of the whole breast). There are small studies suggesting that even lumpectomy alone, without radiation therapy, yields equal survival rates for this type of cancer. But bigger, longer-term studies are needed to confirm this.

It's important for there to be good communication between you and your radiologist after a lumpectomy is done for DCIS. For example, you should have a follow-up mammogram after lumpectomy surgery to be sure no residual calcium was left behind—if your DCIS was associated with calcium.

Mastectomy is still used for larger, more extensive DCIS, or if DCIS is accompanied by diffuse, suspicious microcalcifications in the breast, and your doctor just can't biopsy them all, mastectomy may be recommended. (If a mastectomy is done, radiation is not needed for DCIS.) Because there is only a 1–3 percent chance of having positive lymph nodes associated with DCIS, it is quite rare for the lymph nodes to be removed in

Ductal Carcinoma-in-Situ

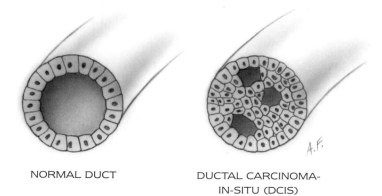

NORMAL DUCT   DUCTAL CARCINOMA-
IN-SITU (DCIS)

treating this condition. If lymph nodes are involved with DCIS, there is probably some invasive component to this cancer that has been missed. But a new treatment, known as sentinel node biopsy, may be used in women with extensive DCIS (that is, large or aggressive tumors). Sentinel node biopsy is discussed more fully on page 176.

Finally, you do *not* need chemotherapy to treat DCIS. Hot off the press right now is the fact that tamoxifen may be useful either in treating DCIS to cut the risk of recurrence, or to reduce the risk of cancer in the opposite breast.

Is it just me, or do we *really* need a song here?

**To the tune of
"We Go Together" from *Grease***

Go check your boobies
Get a mamma, mamma, mamma, a mamma mamm mammogram
You'll feel so groovy
It's better than gettin' a super-size candy gram!
You can . . . even take a buddy
Someone to hold your hand
Isn't that grand!

The doctor does the test
She's gonna squoosh your breast
Between the cool machine
Won't take long, hope you hear
There was no cause to fear
Your breasts are cancer-clean!

Mamma mamma mamma, a mammogram for you
It is the healthful, prudent thing to do
Ring ring, call the doc today
Set the time and get there right away
Boobedy, boobedy, boobedy, boobedy, ba-boob ba-boob ka-boob
Checkity checkity checkity checkity check, ka-check ka-check
Do a lot for your life and your boobity-boobs!
Go!

A second type of in-situ breast condition is known as LCIS, or lobular carcinoma-in-situ. Actually, LCIS is not a "real" cancer. But it does suggest an increased risk for developing a future cancer, and should be taken seriously. If a cancer develops, it does so with equal frequency in both breasts, so in days past, we used to do double mastectomies (remove both breasts) in women with LCIS. We now know that watchful waiting is often a better course. Instead of operating, we usually follow patients closely with careful mammograms and physical examinations of the breasts. And we also give the option of going on tamoxifen, the hormonal treatment that reduces the risk of breast cancer in women at increased risk of getting it. The risk of LCIS associated with into invasive cancer is between 20 and 30 percent over fifteen to twenty-five years. If you have a family history of breast cancer, this risk is compounded. Only in the rare case does it make sense to perform preventive mastectomies. A new study (called the STAR trial) will look at tamoxifen (Nolvadex) versus raloxifene (Evista), and will look at reducing the risk of developing an invasive cancer in high-risk women (particularly those with a history of LCIS).

WHAT'S THE DIFFERENCE IN THE TREATMENT OF INVASIVE OR INFILTRATING BREAST CANCERS?

Invasive cancers have spread outside of their original location in the breast—perhaps further into the breast itself or maybe outside the breast. Because invasive cancers have the potential to spread to the lymph nodes and to other sites in the body, it is important to look at the lymph nodes and to "stage" the cancer—so this is one important difference in treatment from "in-situ" cancers.

The goal of treatment is to remove the tumor plus a rim of healthy surrounding tissue. Radiation therapy is often used after surgery. Mastectomy, removal of the whole breast, is an alternative to lumpectomy plus radiation.

If the tumor is larger than 1 centimeter, our attention turns to chemotherapy, or anticancer drug treatment—another big difference from the treatment of in-situ cancers. About 30 percent of women with negative lymph nodes (that is, nodes clear of cancer) will still go on to have distant cancer, in the bones, lungs, brain, or liver, for example. The remaining 70 percent will have no distant spread. What this means, obviously, is that we may unnecessarily treat 7 out of 10 women with chemotherapy drugs—but we simply cannot predict whose cancer will spread and whose will not. This is when choices about treatment become more complicated, and it becomes important to weigh the risks of chemotherapy treatment against its benefits. For instance, a young woman who is still menstruating runs the chance of going into menopause as a result of chemotherapy. And certain chemotherapeutic drugs can themselves cause blood cancers. These and other risks and side effects must be weighed against the potential benefits these drugs can offer in your fight against breast cancer. You must ask your doctor what your expected survival advantage is, given your age and particular breast cancer stage, before choosing a treatment regimen.

WHAT IS THIS NEW TECHNIQUE I'M HEARING ABOUT CALLED SENTINEL NODE BIOPSY?

The sentinel node biopsy marks one of the great achievements in the fight against breast cancer, and a potential revolution in how the disease will be surgically treated. As I discussed earlier, in some cases we have to take out a woman's lymph nodes to see if cancer has spread there. This process can lead to a serious problem, known as lymphedema, which I will explain in more detail in a moment. With lymphedema, there may be severe swelling in the arm after removal of the lymph nodes. But sentinel node biopsy helps do away with this problem.

It works as follows:

Instead of going in and taking out a whole bunch of lymph nodes, we take some interesting steps to remove just one or two so-called sentinel nodes—which you can think of as the guards or leaders of the lymph nodes. These guardian nodes are re-

---

CANCER STAGING TABLE

STAGE 0:

Noninvasive or in-situ breast cancer. The cancer cells are limited to the ducts or lobules in the breast, and have not penetrated the walls of these structures.
DCIS (intraductal cancer or ductal carcinoma-in-situ).
LCIS (lobular carcinoma-in-situ); although it is called "cancer," we regard LCIS as a precancerous lesion, or a marker for breast cancer.

STAGE 1:

The tumor is equal to or smaller than 2 centimeters (about ¾ inch), and has not spread beyond the breast.

STAGE 2 (MAY BE DIVIDED INTO 2A AND 2B):

The tumor is larger than 2 centimeters and/or lymph nodes under the arm are positive for cancer. (Note: This stage does *not* mean that cancer has definitely spread to the lymph nodes.)

STAGE 3—DIVIDED INTO 3A AND 3B:

3A—The tumor is larger than 5 centimeters (two inches) in diameter and has spread to the lymph nodes.
3B—The tumor spreads to the skin, chest wall, or lymph nodes near the breastbone. For example, inflammatory cancer is considered stage 3B.

STAGE 4:

Cancer that has spread to other distant sites in the body, e.g., the bones, lungs, brain, or liver.

---

sponsible for draining the cancerous tumor, and are thought to represent the first "stop" on the cancer's travels through the lymph system. By injecting a radioactive substance and/or a blue dye, we can now trace the tumor's drainage system and find the sentinel node(s). The radioactive material and dye literally drain through the lymph system and then "light up" the node(s) in question. You can think of this like the metal detectors people drag along the beach in search of lost coins. When I find that "hot" node, I know I've struck treasure.

This is a very operator-dependent process, and there is a steep learning curve, so your doctor should base decisions on it only if he or she is confident that the results have been reliable in his or her hands. Once we find the sentinel node(s), we immediately do a so-called frozen section to study it for cancer. If the node is found to be cancer-free, your doctor can stop there. We still send the node(s) for special testing, however, because about 1 out of 10 times, more sensitive testing does reveal some cancer in the node(s), which we consider evidence of "micrometastasis"—or tiny cancer spread. If the sentinel node is found positive for cancer, then another surgery is required and a standard node dissection is done. I cannot stress how valuable it is to be able to avoid so many node dissections and thereby avert the terrible complications that can result from them.

◆ Why is this so important?

Because we have learned that if the sentinel node(s) is free of cancer, we can expect that the other nodes are free of cancer as well. And if we can avoid removing all of those other nodes, we can help women avoid the most feared complication of breast cancer surgery—lymphedema, or severe arm swelling, which can be permanent and terribly debilitating.

Now, sentinel node biopsy is not for everyone. If your doctor actually feels on a physical examination that your underarm lymph nodes are swollen and are likely positive for cancer, then a sentinel node biopsy will not be done. The traditional removal of several lymph nodes will be needed instead. Other cases in which you should *not* do sentinel node biopsy include: (1) very large tumors; (2) more than one tumor, at different sites in the breast, known as "multicentricity"; (3) when preoperative chemotherapy was given; (4) prior axillary (underarm) surgery; or (5) pregnancy.

Most *major* treatment centers now offer sentinel node

biopsy, but relatively few doctors around the country are trained to do it. This will likely change as more women demand the procedure.

◆ CAN I BE TREATED FOR BREAST CANCER DURING PREGNANCY?

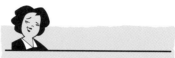

As a breast surgeon, my primary concern is the health of the mother, though certainly our goal is to protect the health of both mother and baby. But there are many different scenarios to consider. For instance, if invasive breast cancer is found

Yes. Just think, morning sickness throughout the day.

early in the pregnancy, mastectomy is recommended as part of treatment, because it is simply too dangerous for an early-stage fetus to be exposed to radiation treatments. If breast cancer is found later in pregnancy, even a month before delivery, then we will often go ahead and do lumpectomy surgery on the woman while she is pregnant, and then wait until after delivery to do the radiation therapy. Chemotherapy is a different story, which I will discuss shortly.

Naturally, we take special precautions during surgery on a pregnant woman—such as extra care with anesthesia, and special positioning of the mother in order to reduce pressure on the main vein that supplies blood to the uterus. We are also especially careful about controlling bleeding, since the breasts are rich with blood vessels at this time, as the body anticipates breast-feeding. If I operate on someone who is breast-feeding, I ask her to continue to feed the baby or to pump her milk shortly afterward. You can pump out your first milk after surgery to get rid of the residual anesthetic. But the idea is to get the milk out of the breast so it doesn't build up and force its way through your surgical incision, causing a "milk fistula." Milk also happens to be a great medium for bacteria to grow in, so ask your doctor for antibiotics around the time of surgery to help you avoid mastitis (a breast infection). The bottom line, however, is that despite these various concerns and subsequent precautions, you want to have treatment for breast cancer ASAP. Don't let breast-feeding, or pregnancy for that matter, delay treatments that can save your life. Chemotherapy is another issue in pregnancy. Some drugs are considered relatively safe for the developing fetus, while others would be too toxic. This is something to discuss with your doctor.

Much more complex emotional and philosophical questions come into play as well. For example, you have to think very carefully about bringing a new life into the world if, for example, your prognosis is not good. What support systems are in place for the baby if you are not able to care for it? What, if any, is the decrease in your survival chances if you go through with the pregnancy? Do you have other young children who need your care? These enormously serious and painful questions cannot be worked out with your medical doctors alone. This is a time when other support people, including loved ones, social workers and other therapists, and spiritual advisers like clergy can help you sort out your feelings and priorities. Talking to other women who have gone through the same experience can help as well—you can often get phone numbers from your doctor. Ultimately, of course, these critical decisions will be your own. But the more support you can garner in making them, the easier the load on your shoulders—which are already bearing quite a burden.

◆ CAN I BECOME PREGNANT AFTER BEING TREATED FOR BREAST CANCER?

Yes. However, there *is* a risk of going into early menopause after taking some anticancer drugs. The younger you are, the lower the risk of losing your fertility due to breast cancer treatments. One somewhat reassuring study has found that

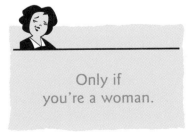

Only if
you're a woman.

among women treated with a common breast cancer drug regimen CMF (for cyclophosphamide, methotrexate, and 5-fluorouracil), the risk of ovarian failure is 0 percent for women under thirty years of age; 33 percent for women aged thirty to thirty-nine; 96 percent for those forty to forty-nine; and 100 percent only for those over fifty, who have almost reached the average age of natural menopause anyway.

Studies have shown that if you still ovulate after breast cancer treatment, you can successfully carry a pregnancy. (Some studies have even found a better prognosis among women who become pregnant after breast cancer, but this could be a result of the fact that women with earlier cancers are more likely to become pregnant.) Since it is known that invasive breast cancer recurrence is most likely in the first two years after treatment, I urge women to wait two to three years to become pregnant after treatment. But talk to your doctor about your own particular case.

◆ CAN I BREAST-FEED AFTER BREAST CANCER?

If your surgery and/or radiation treatment did not interfere with your milk production (by creating a mechanical blockage so that the milk cannot travel through your nipples), you can, technically, still breast-feed. But there may be some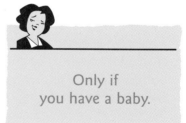

Only if
you have a baby.

complications. For instance, if you develop an infection in your breast during breast-feeding (known as a mastitis), it would be harder to treat because of the inner scarring from more extensive surgery and/or radiation treatment. A major infection would be hard to treat with antibiotics and it would be more difficult to fully empty the breast of milk, which is important in the treatment of mastitis. You could, therefore, end up with an abscess (a cavity filled with pus).

If you are seriously committed to breast-feeding, however, there are some solutions. For example, you can breast-feed from one breast (and not from the breast formerly treated for cancer). This might not be cosmetically ideal, since the breast filled with milk can appear much larger than the other breast. Because some women already have disproportionate breasts after cancer treatment, this might be additionally awkward. But it is one option for women who want very much to breast-feed.

There are other important issues to keep in mind as well. For instance, it is harder to physically examine a lactating breast—and it's also harder to image a lactating breast with tools such as the mammogram. Since women who have undergone breast cancer often need careful follow-up, this can complicate matters. The breast can take as long as two years to get back to its resting state after pregnancy and breast-feeding, and because mammography is seldom done during pregnancy, this means that a great deal of time can add up between mammograms. Sometimes, I'll see a woman who is extremely dedicated to breast-feeding but absolutely needs a follow-up mammogram. What I do is ask her to bring the baby to the mammography center and feed him until the breast is soft, not engorged; then I do one X-ray view of each breast instead of the standard two or more views. If the image is too obscured, you can stop right there instead of doing more. If the breast is filled with milk, there's no point doing the mammogram. Unless there is some important reason to do otherwise (e.g., if I am following up on calcium deposits), I usually like to wait four to six months after the completion of breast-feeding to do a mammogram.

◆ IS THERE ANY RISK THAT THE BABY WILL GET RADIATION IN THE MILK AFTER A MAMMOGRAM?

We don't know if the baby would get any radiation at all, or even if it did, if that would pose any problems. However, a good way to feel more secure is to empty your breast of milk using some other means (a breast pump, for example) after the mammogram. Then, "fresh" milk will fill the breast for the baby's next feeding.

WHEN YOU TREAT BREAST CANCER, DO YOU TREAT OLDER WOMEN AND YOUNGER WOMEN ANY DIFFERENTLY?

Yes.
We talk louder to
the older women.

Treatment differences are not determined by age per se, but there happen to be some differences in the types of cancers occurring in older and younger women, and this does affect treatment. But certainly given the same type and degree of cancer, treatment should be the same regardless of age.

For a long time, people made the terrible error of assuming that there was little value in saving the breasts of older women—who allegedly "didn't need them" anymore. The callous presumption was that older women no longer need their breasts for breast-feeding, nor do they need them for sexuality or femininity. Nothing could be further from the truth. I feel that largely *because* older age is a time when women's bodies change—the breasts and skin sag, muscle tone weakens, vaginal lubrication lessens, and so on—it is especially critical to save any element of sexuality and femininity possible. Self-image is every bit as important—if not more so—than it was in women's youth. So older women should be educated, just as younger women should be, about the option to save their breasts and elect the lumpectomy procedure instead of mastectomy. That said, there are certain cases in which much older, generally weak or unhealthy women may not be eligible for aspects of treatment that require regular attendance at the doctor's office. For instance, radiation therapy may not be possible for a woman who cannot function without professional assistance. In this case, lumpectomy plus radiation may not be feasible, and a mastectomy is the better option. Always remember, though, that any *informed* choice is a good choice; even a woman eligible for lumpectomy who chooses mastectomy after carefully considering her options is doing the "right thing" for herself. Choosing among options is empowering for women of all ages and profiles.

Where should I go for breast cancer treatment?

Certainly you want a center of excellence, but such excellence can come in different guises. For example, while it is critically important to have a strong and communicative cancer-fighting team (including a surgeon, radiologist, pathologist,

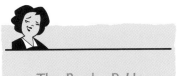

The Boobs R Us drive-thru.

radiation oncologist, medical oncologist, social workers, nurses, and so on), there are also superb individual doctors in private offices who offer the best of care. The question is, if you've found someone good who practices independently, does that person have connections and regular interaction with other cancer care specialists? Can he or she work as part of a team? This is extremely important.

You want to find doctors who are busy and active treating patients with conditions similar to yours. I personally would rather see a lesser-known surgeon who has done a thousand procedures similar to the one I need and who regularly attends all of the main conferences and continuing education in the field, than a big-name doctor who spends less time treating patients and more time on the lecture circuit.

If you want to find a center of excellence, there are a few ways to go about doing so. First, the National Cancer Institute designates a number of so-called comprehensive cancer care centers around the country, as well as several community hospitals and centers worthy of note. (You can find a list of the NCI-designated centers on pages 281–90.) And the American College of Surgeons accredits cancer centers as well.

If I have cancer in one breast, should I have the other one treated as well?

About ½ to 1 percent of breast cancer survivors per year (15 percent over a lifetime) have a second breast cancer in the opposite breast. These are not huge numbers. As a result, I usually don't recommend removing the other breast "just as a precaution." I prefer to have patients carefully monitored with frequent mammograms and physical examinations. Also, with the use of the hormonal drug tamoxifen, we can reduce a high-risk woman's chance of developing a cancer in her healthy breast by nearly 50 percent—and that's a big number. The combination of vigilant screening and, if appropriate, tamoxifen therapy is usually preferable to removing a healthy breast.

If you have had breast cancer yourself and also have a significant family history of the disease, I recommend that you sit down with a genetic counselor to discuss your risk, and possibly undergo genetic testing in order to determine if you carry a breast cancer gene. This helps us to determine just how great your personal risk actually is. The more you know about your own particular case, the easier it is to make treatment—and "prevention"—choices.

◆ MY BREAST CANCER WAS CAUGHT VERY EARLY. DO I NEED CHEMOTHERAPY?

Cancer-fighting drugs are not used in women with noninvasive breast cancers. However, we do know that even in early, *invasive* node-negative breast cancer, there is a 30 percent chance of developing a distant spread of the cancer. For this reason, in women with tumors that appear to be aggressive, or whose tumors are larger than 1 centimeter in size, we may offer chemotherapy even with negative nodes. But we stress the fact that the improvement in survival rates is quite small, and that it's vital to compare the small increased survival benefit with the risks and side effects of the treatment itself.

◆ Does the timing of my breast cancer surgery matter?

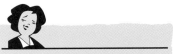

The sooner you operate, the better—because delays in treatment
give cancer time to spread. That
said, there is some interesting evidence that operating at different
times in a woman's menstrual cycle
may influence survival rates. It has

Yes. Do it in the morning so you don't miss *General Hospital.*

been shown in some studies that when tumors are removed
during the luteal phase of the menstrual cycle—that is, on days
0 through 2 and days 13 through 32 of the cycle—the prognosis is better than when tumors are removed in the follicular
phase (days 3 through 12).

There are several theories as to why this might be true, including the fact that there is a possible increase in natural killer
cells in the body during the luteal phase of the menstrual cycle.
But I always tell my patients—especially those with erratic
menstrual cycles—that if you spend too much time waiting for
the alleged "right" time to operate, you may just wait too long
and risk hurting your prognosis because of the delay. Keep in
mind that some of these studies were rather imprecise, in that
they failed to measure accurately the blood levels of estrogen at
each supposed point in the menstrual cycle. So what I recommend is that if a woman has very regular cycles, and it's easy to
determine the various stages of those cycles and to schedule
breast cancer surgery accordingly, by all means do it. If, on the
other hand, it is going to take up lots of time and create confu-
sion trying to match the surgery to some point in the cycle, it
may not be worth the delay.

◆ Is the treatment of breast cancer standard throughout the United States?

Far from it. Several studies have shown that where you live has a direct impact on the kind of breast cancer treatment you will be offered—and receive. For example, it has been shown that women who live in the South are less likely to get the breast-sparing lumpectomy procedure (37.8 percent) than women who live in the Northeast (61.4 percent). This is not ex-

> Some people prefer standard, and some people prefer automatic. If you ask me, stick shifts are always tough.

plained by the fact that women in the South have more extensive disease. For some, the choice of mastectomy is due to inaccessibility of radiation facilities. Also, doctors in some areas have more conservative biases about treatment, and because removal of the breast was the old-line treatment for breast cancer, they've stuck with that recommendation. Women in some regions of the country may not be informed of their surgical and other treatment options, and therefore have more old-fashioned biases about how to treat the disease (or just don't know what questions to ask about it). A relatively high percentage of *older* women still have mastectomy, which could reflect that ageism is present in medical care in parts of the country—i.e., doctors thinking "She's old, what does she need her breasts for?" This is a terrible fallacy.

Ethnicity also seems to play a big role in breast cancer treatment. Caucasian women, for example, are more likely to have modern, breast-conserving procedures than are Native American women. This could be a combination of differences in education and also a reflection of the lack of adequate widespread screening in some populations, which results in more advanced cancers and, in turn, more extensive treatments. Also, income plays a role: Women from higher socioeconomic groups tend to have more treatment choices (57.4 percent) than those from less affluent backgrounds (41.4 percent). Clearly there is some interface between income, education, and exposure to the most current breast cancer treatment options. Finally, young African American women have a disproportionately high risk of dying from breast cancer when compared to Caucasian women. This may partially reflect inadequate breast screening in this population, which results in cancers being detected later, when they are more serious and harder to cure.

The lesson that should come out of this, for all women, is that we can count on no one but ourselves to gather the information needed to make smart breast cancer treatment choices. The many resources listed at the end of this book offer free, accessible information on every aspect of breast cancer diagnosis, treatment, and aftercare for women of every background and experience.

◆ I'VE HEARD THAT SOME WOMEN CAN BE TREATED AS PART OF SCIENTIFIC STUDIES OR CLINICAL TRIALS. WHAT DOES THIS MEAN?

Clinical trials are studies, with several phases, that evaluate a given treatment for a certain type of disease. The researchers who conduct clinical trials follow a carefully designed treatment plan called a protocol. This spells out what will be done, and why. In the first phase of a clinical trial, researchers look for a

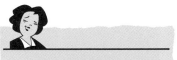

It means that some women can be treated as part of scientific studies or clinical trials.

safe and well-tolerated dose of the given drug. In the second phase, they try to identify tumor types for which the treatment might be most promising. In the third phase, they compare the new treatment to another standard treatment for the disease.

Usually, there are strict requirements to be included in a clinical trial—such as a particular stage of disease, type of tumor, perhaps your age or some other criteria, and so on. You will need to have a complete, detailed diagnosis of your type of breast cancer. To find out if you are eligible for a clinical trial, you can contact the National Cancer Institute (NCI). The NCI has a brochure entitled "What Are Clinical Trials All About: A Booklet for Patients with Cancer." The American Society of Clinical Oncologists (ASCO) also has a pamphlet about volunteering for a clinical trial.

Your doctor does *not* need to be part of a well-known cancer center in order for you to participate in a clinical trial. However, it is important that he or she knows how to affiliate with a larger center, or with a National Institutes of Health trial, so that you can take part in such a study.

♦ THESE DAYS YOU READ SO MUCH ABOUT THE USE OF ALTERNATIVE AND COMPLEMENTARY MEDICINE. DO THESE APPROACHES PLAY A ROLE IN THE TREATMENT OF BREAST CANCER?

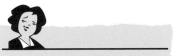

In short, yes—but this depends a great deal on where you live, your health care practitioner's attitudes toward these therapies, and other related factors. Before I talk about the role of alternative and complementary medicine in the treatment of breast cancer, though, let me spend a minute differentiating the

Sorry, the question is too long and I dozed off in the middle.

two. Alternative medicine refers to nonconventional, unproved treatments for the cancer itself. These are treatments usually recommended *instead* of conventional cancer therapies. Some common alternative therapies for breast cancer include the Revici Method, the Gerson Method, high-dose intravenous vitamin therapy, the macrobiotic diet, the Contrarist Method—and this is only the tip of the iceberg. Complementary therapies, on the other hand, are treatments that are recommended for use *in conjunction with* mainstream cancer treatments. Complementary therapies are not intended to treat the cancer itself, but to help heal the whole person with cancer. These therapies include massage, relaxation therapy, nutritional support, yoga, visualization, guided imagery, aromatherapy, acupuncture, and many other related approaches.

While I am leery about alternative therapies (they are often recommended by destructive practitioners who wrongly label chemotherapy as a "poison"), I am extremely happy to see that the use of complementary therapies is on the increase. At the Geffen Cancer Center and Research Institute in Vero Beach, Florida, for example, an impressive program has been developed where the most effective mainstream cancer treatments are blended with a rainbow of the best complementary therapies available. Patients are massaged before receiving chemotherapy in order to reduce both their stress levels and their side effects from treatment. Patients sleep better, have better digestion, and feel relaxed despite the physical and emotional toll of treatment. They listen to relaxing music during chemotherapy. They take classes in deep breathing and other powerful stress-reduction techniques. They learn to visualize the death of their cancer cells. And much more. The guiding concept here is that you don't just treat the cancer, you treat the *person* with cancer—and this requires attention to the heart, mind, body, and spirit.

Do complementary therapies help fight the cancer as well? That's debatable. There are studies suggesting that massage, for example, can help raise various immune factors in the body and thereby help fight cancer cells. If this is true, then all the better. But I would argue that even if complementary therapies do nothing more than make women with breast cancer feel better in the here and now, they should be applauded and encouraged.

Now, the story is less cheery when it comes to the use of various herbal therapies, which are sometimes part of complementary and alternative treatment for cancer. While there are some very good reasons to use some herbal remedies—for instance, in the treatment of menopausal symptoms that arise after chemotherapy—it is not always safe to take herbs while undergoing other conventional treatments for cancer. Herbal preparations often contain hundreds of ingredients, few if any of which have been studied for their effects when interacting with conventional cancer drugs. One worrisome example would be the use of coenzyme 10, the antioxidant that some practitioners recommend for use along with chemotherapy or radiation therapy. There is some evidence that this treatment can undermine the effectiveness of the cancer treatments. Or, as another example, herbal preparations like ginseng or dong quoi can contain large amounts of the hormone estrogen—which can fuel some breast cancers. For these and other reasons, I strongly advise those of you who are considering using herbal therapies during or shortly after chemotherapy to discuss the issue thoroughly with your doctor.

As always, however, the ultimate goal of cancer therapy is customization. Just as a given conventional treatment may not be advisable in your case, so a complementary therapy may be right for one woman, and not for you. Whatever your treatment choices, be sure that your doctors have excellent and clearly spelled-out reasons why they are appropriate for your particular cancer—and for your particular body. And if you are selecting treatments from different "families" of therapy, be sure that your doctor is carefully orchestrating your care so that both conventional and complementary treatments are safe and suited to one another.

TREATMENT

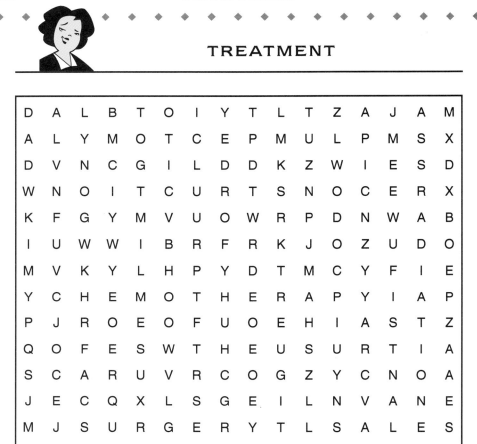

D	A	L	B	T	O	I	Y	T	L	T	Z	A	J	A	M
A	L	Y	M	O	T	C	E	P	M	U	L	P	M	S	X
D	V	N	C	G	I	L	D	D	K	Z	W	I	E	S	D
W	N	O	I	T	C	U	R	T	S	N	O	C	E	R	X
K	F	G	Y	M	V	U	O	W	R	P	D	N	W	A	B
I	U	W	W	I	B	R	F	R	K	J	O	Z	U	D	O
M	V	K	Y	L	H	P	Y	D	T	M	C	Y	F	I	E
Y	C	H	E	M	O	T	H	E	R	A	P	Y	I	A	P
P	J	R	O	E	O	F	U	O	E	H	I	A	S	T	Z
Q	O	F	E	S	W	T	H	E	U	S	U	R	T	I	A
S	C	A	R	U	V	R	C	O	G	Z	Y	C	N	O	A
J	E	C	Q	X	L	S	G	E	I	L	N	V	A	N	E
M	J	S	U	R	G	E	R	Y	T	L	S	A	L	E	S
C	Z	E	H	H	Y	S	S	B	A	S	M	T	P	V	U
B	S	S	E	N	D	L	A	B	F	J	A	U	M	W	A
B	H	A	M	E	D	E	H	P	M	Y	L	M	I	E	N

Find and circle the following words:

BALDNESS	LUMPECTOMY	RADIATION
CHEMOTHERAPY	LYMPHEDEMA	RECONSTRUCTION
FATIGUE	MASTECTOMY	SCAR
HORMONES	NAUSEA	SURGERY
IMPLANTS		

6

AFTERCARE:
Life after Breast Cancer

LINDA ELLERBEE

I remember back in the beginning, right after I'd found out the terrible news, a friend who's HIV-positive told me there would be positive things that would come to me because I had a life-threatening disease. I remember laughing at him. Better living through cancer? Puleeze.

Today I begin to understand how right he was. In my case, that's made easier by the fact that now, I am by all tests clear of cancer.

I am also happier than I've ever been in my life.

What? You have no breasts, you say?

True, but look what I do have.

I'm alive.

I have, in fact, never been quite so alive. Or so healthy. I quit smoking. I bike fifteen miles a day. I walk. I hike. I work out. I sweat. I eat fruit and vegetables and fish, and drink gallons of water. I feel absolutely wonderful. I have the energy of women half my age. And I go around saying "thank you" a lot. Like all the time. Everyday life seems to me now to be a great, good gift, and I'm a healthy, happy, grateful woman. Ain't that enough?

I know, breasts are a big deal in America, but well, so what. Breathing is a big deal, too, and I'm still breathing. And raising hell.

IMMEDIATE AFTERCARE:

◆ HOW SHOULD I CARE FOR MY WOUND AFTER BREAST SURGERY?

If all goes properly, you shouldn't *have* to care for your wound—your doctor should do that for you with proper dressings and so on. Ask your doctor whether he or she uses dissolving stitches, for example, which allow you to avoid a return visit for suture removal. And request a special kind of plastic dressing on the wound that will enable you to take a shower right away. Many women crave a good, deep-cleansing shower after surgery.

The only real work that should be required of you after mastectomy surgery is care of your drain. You'll have to learn how to empty the drain, how to keep the bulb on suction so that it will continue to take fluid out from under your arm or from the mastectomy flaps. Make sure your doctor gives you a good long tube so that you can empty the drain yourself—if it's too short, this can be difficult. Maintenance of your drain should be fully explained to you until you are comfortable with the device. Problem signs to watch for include bright red drainage, which can indicate bleeding in and around the drain, and redness where the drain exits your body, which can indicate an infection. Generally the drain is clipped to the inside of your clothing, but I strongly recommend a fanny pack to hold the drain so you can wander around and remain mobile. Also be sure to request enough gauze and tape to reapply around your drain after you shower. And keep both a measuring cup and a record of how much fluid is coming from the drain each day, as you can stop using the drain when less than 30 cubic centimeters of fluid (a little more than half a teaspoon) emerges in a twenty-four-hour period. This usually takes between three and seven days.

If you are scared even to look at your surgical wound, you're not alone; many women fear this first glimpse of their newly changed bodies. If you're worried and want to know what to expect, ask your doctor for pictures of other women—but be sure to look at photos of women both immediately after surgery *and* long after recovery, so that you can see the great results that can emerge over time.

◆ WHAT SHOULD I EXPECT AFTER BREAST RECONSTRUCTION SURGERY?

That depends on the type of reconstruction you have done, how your doctor dresses your wounds, and so on. After the TRAM-flap procedure, for example, it's important not to put undue stress on your abdomen for at least a month—but many motivated women are able to exercise again after a month to six weeks. After a reconstruction with implants, the recovery and return to exercise is usually much quicker. Ask your doctor to take you through the specific postsurgical care for your type of reconstruction.

◆ THE AREA OVER MY SURGICAL INCISION IS VERY ITCHY. IS THIS NORMAL?

Yes, and it's a common part of the healing process, which is exacerbated because the wound can't breathe under all that dressing. This feeling should lessen with time.

◆ HOW CAN I LESSEN THE APPEARANCE OF MY SURGICAL SCARS?

If your scars harden, you can help a great deal by massaging them twice a day, for five minutes each session, using some kind of lotion such as cocoa butter, vitamin E cream or oil from vitamin E capsules, or aloe. Use the flat part of your fingers in a back-and-forth walking motion over the scars (do not abrade

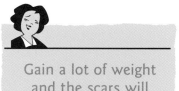

Gain a lot of weight and the scars will look smaller.

◆   ◆   ◆   ◆   ◆   ◆   ◆   ◆   ◆   ◆   ◆   ◆   ◆   ◆   ◆   ◆   ◆

your skin!). Both the scars and the breast should become softer
as a result of these self-administered massage treatments.

◆ **I AM EXPERIENCING TERRIBLE SWELLING IN THE ARM
WHERE MY LYMPH NODES WERE REMOVED. WHAT'S
THE CAUSE AND WHAT CAN I DO ABOUT IT?**

The cause is most likely lymphedema, which refers to fluid
buildup in the arm after lymph
node removal. It develops when
fluid in the arm gets trapped in the
postsurgical scar tissue and cannot
flow back into the blood vessels to

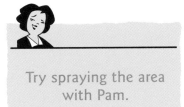

Try spraying the area
with Pam.

be drained away from the arm. It can be mild or severe, and can
appear quickly after surgery or not for many years afterward.
Lymphedema is more than a cosmetic problem, although
women suffer greatly from the unpleasant appearance of a
large, swollen arm. This condition also creates great dysfunc-
tion, with trouble moving and using the affected arm, hardening of the skin of the arm, and other related problems. I had a
patient once who suffered terribly because *his* lymphedema
made it impossible for *him* to do something as simple as toss a
ball to his grandson. Yes, men do get breast cancer—see page
18 for a discussion of this subject.

What causes lymphedema? It is more likely to occur:

- In heavier women;
- When there is a postoperative infection;
- When there are lots of cancer-positive lymph nodes;
- When you receive postoperative radiation therapy (which
is done rarely when lymph nodes are being removed); and
- When there is "excessive dissection" (that is, large
amounts of surgery and disruption in the armpit).

It is always important for your doctor to rule out other
problems that might be causing arm swelling (such as a recur-

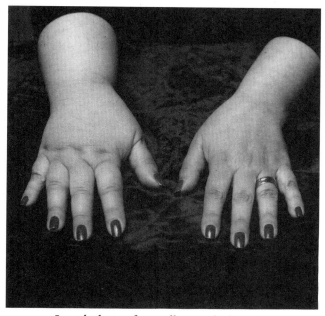

Lymphedema after axillary node dissection.
Rings and other constricting jewelry should be avoided
on the affected side.

rent tumor, vascular problems—such as a blood clot—an underlying infection, or heart problems). To be absolutely sure there's no hidden infection, I give my patients a course of antibiotics for a week or so before I further treat the lymphedema.

If you are diagnosed with lymphedema, however, there are several steps you can take to control it. The condition is not considered "curable," but it is manageable. First, you must be fitted for a compression garment or sleeve to compress the arm and help keep it from retaining fluid. *Do not buy such a garment over the counter.* It is extremely important to have a proper fitting so that the compression is just right for you. The compression is measured in millimeters of mercury, and should be customized to your particular case. You don't need to wear the sleeve all the time—six hours a day would be good. Many women are bothered by the appearance of the sleeve—so I always tell my patients they don't need to wear it to dinner. Do not wear the sleeve to bed, as lymphedema tends to lessen overnight because of the elevated position of the arm during sleep. Also, when watching TV or relaxing, keep your arm elevated on top of two pillows. And by the way—for the small number of women who are allergic to the material in most compression sleeves, there are alternatives, so ask for a different material.

You should also learn a number of arm and hand protection methods, including the following:

- If you garden, use canvas gloves.
- Use rubber gloves when cleaning with steel wool, hot water, or harsh detergents.
- Wear long (elbow-length) oven mitts when cooking or working near heat.
- Don't cut your cuticles, to avoid infection—and be careful with manicures.
- Don't wear restrictive clothing (too-tight bra straps, for example) or accessories such as a tight wristwatch, ring, or bracelet.
- Don't wear a too-heavy breast prosthesis—ask your doctor for guidance.
- If you sew, use a thimble to protect you from cuts.
- If you have a heavy purse, don't carry it on the arm with lymphedema.
- Avoid heavy lifting in general.
- Use common sense with exercise—for example, three-pound weights may be fine, but very heavy ones are not recommended.
- Wear your compression sleeve during exercise or essential heavy work.
- Avoid having your blood pressure taken in the affected arm.
- Avoid injections in the affected arm.
- Avoid excessive sun exposure, which can cause burns and, in turn, more swelling.

• Avoid extreme temperature changes, including very hot baths, hot tubs, showers, and saunas, and travel in excessively hot climates (and any other source of burns, including smoking).

• Some say to avoid salt in the diet and to use diuretics, but this is controversial, so ask your own doctor's opinion on it.

• Be very careful when shaving your underarm, to avoid cuts.

• Avoid insect bites and animal bites and scratches.

• Keep your weight in check: obesity greatly increases the risk of lymphedema.

Finally, an important part of lymphedema management—and prevention—is exercise. Proper exercises should be started shortly after the initial operation. I have patients begin these as soon as the drain is removed after surgery. Keep in mind that any exercise program needs to be customized after breast reconstruction, so discuss this issue with both your breast surgeon and your plastic surgeon, if you have one. For instance, exercises with continued rapid, repetitive motion can worsen, rather than lessen, lymphedema. (In the old days, we had to recommend more formal physical therapy after lymph node removal, because of a problem called "frozen shoulder," in which women literally could not move their shoulder or arm after extensive surgery followed by radiation to the underarm area. Today, improved techniques make this type of severe immobility *extremely* rare.)

Here are a few exercises that can help you retain (or regain) good range of motion in the affected arm. If needed, take pain medication about thirty to forty-five minutes before exercising.

◆   ◆   ◆   ◆   ◆   ◆   ◆   ◆   ◆   ◆   ◆   ◆   ◆   ◆   ◆   ◆   ◆   ◆   ◆   ◆

SHOULDER ROLLS
AND NECK EXERCISES

1. Sit up straight in a chair or at the edge of the bed, or stand up straight.

2. Look straight ahead and keep your head up. In one continuous motion, raise both shoulders upward, move them backward and then down, forward and up, and around to the start position. Repeat for 10 circles.

3. Repeat circles, beginning the movement upward, then forward, down, and around. Do 10 forward motion circles.

4. Turn your head to the left so that your nose is over your shoulder. Move your head to the center or start position then turn your head to the right so that your nose is over your shoulder. Return to the center or start position. Repeat 5–10 times.

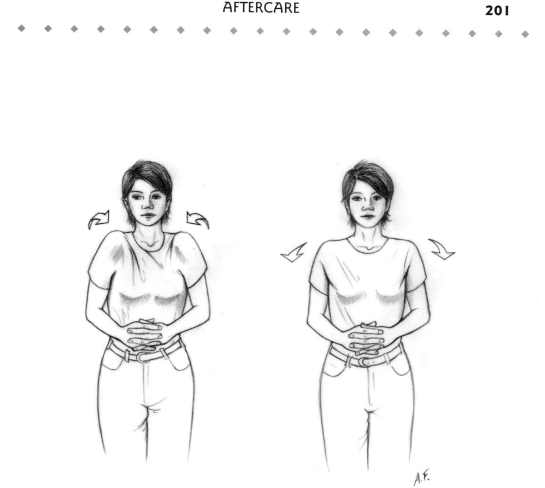

WALL CLIMBING

1. The first time you do this exercise, stand facing the wall with your feet about six inches away from the wall. With the arm on the side that has NOT had surgery, reach as high as you can. Make a mark on the wall with a pencil or piece of tape. This marks your normal range of movement. Your goal is to reach the mark on the wall with the arm on the side that had surgery. If you have had surgery on both sides, you may set your goal with the arm that moves more comfortably.

2. To begin the exercise, face the wall with your feet about six inches away from the wall. Place hands on the wall, shoulder width apart and on the same level with each other. Slowly "walk or crawl" your hands up the wall until you feel incisional pulling or discomfort. Stop and hold this position for one minute. You can use deep breathing to help relieve the pulling. After one minute, slowly crawl your hands up the wall a little bit farther until you feel incisional pulling or discomfort. Hold this position for one minute.

3. After one minute, slowly "crawl" your hand back down the wall until you reach the start position. Do not just drop your hands, because that movement will release the stretch too quickly. Remember, the goal of this exercise is to stretch out the scar tissue. It is the deliberate crawling and holding of the position that will help you reach your goal.

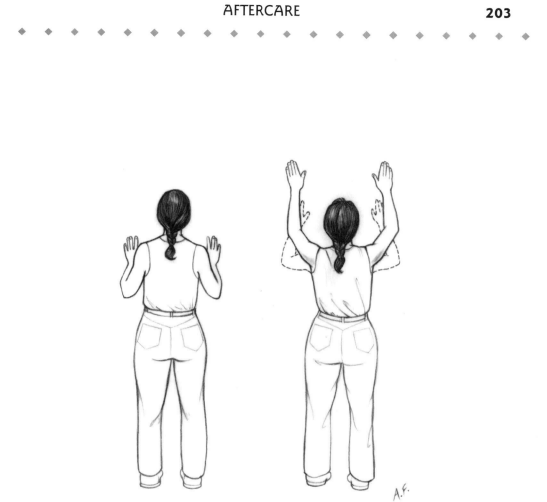

◆ ◆

CLASP, REACH, AND SPREAD

1. Sit up straight in a chair, preferably facing a mirror. Start the exercise with your hands clasped in your lap. The goal is to move your hands all the way to the back of your neck.

2. Slowly raise your hands toward your forehead, keeping your elbows as close together as possible. If you feel incisional pulling or discomfort, stop and rest your hands where they are (your chin, nose, forehead, top of your head) and hold the position for one minute. You may do deep breathing until the pulling subsides. If the pain does not subside, slowly return to the start position after one minute. If it does subside, continue the exercise until you feel the pulling again. Hold for one minute. Then return slowly to the start position. It may take several sessions for you to complete all the positions of this exercise. Take your time, and remember that the goal of stretching is to relax the scar tissue.

3. As you are able to go further with the exercise, slide your hands over your head, keeping your elbows close to your ears. Remember to keep your head up! Check your position to make sure you can see your chin in the mirror. Slide your hands down until they reach the base of your neck. When your hands reach the base of your neck, open your elbows wide out to the side. Hold this position for one minute. Slowly reverse direction and return to the start position.

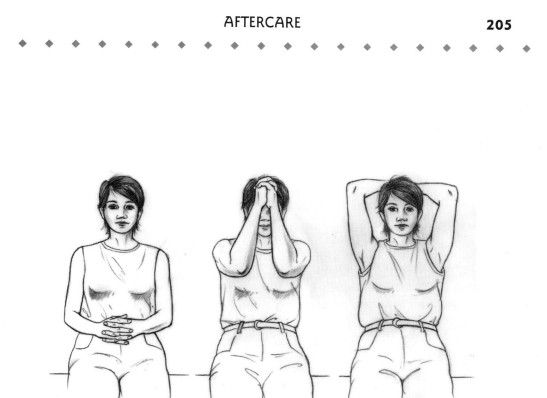

SIDE WALL STRETCH

Once you have reached your full range of motion with the above exercises, this exercise will help you to stretch a little more:

1. Stand perpendicular (sideways) to the wall with the arm on the side of surgery facing the wall and your feet about one foot away from the wall. Reach your arm up to the wall and put the heel of your hand on the wall. Do not rest your weight on your fingers.

2. Lean into the wall so that the heel of your hand slides up the wall until you feel incisional pulling. Hold this position for one minute. Return to the start position.

3. Repeat the exercise until you no longer feel incisional pulling while your arm is at the full height of the position.

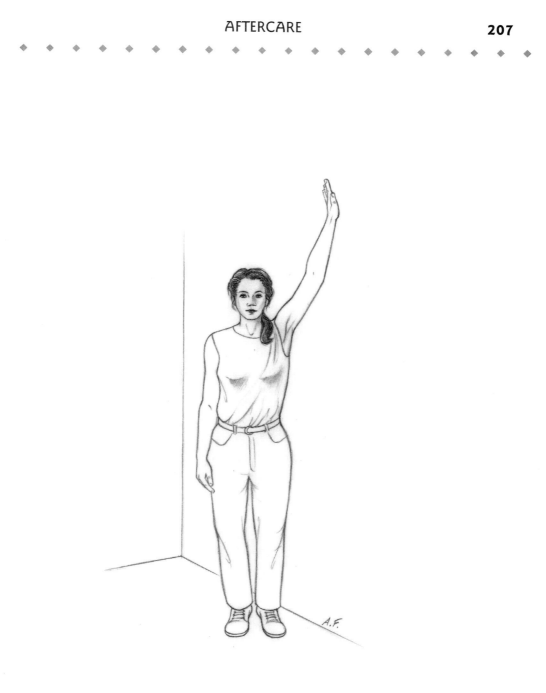

◆ ◆ ◆ ◆ ◆ ◆ ◆ ◆ ◆ ◆ ◆ ◆ ◆ ◆ ◆ ◆ ◆ ◆ ◆ ◆

◆ DOES ANYONE USE PUMPS TO RELIEVE THE SWELLING OF LYMPHEDEMA ANYMORE?

In the past, pumps were used to mechanically push fluid out of the arm with lymphedema. But in a matter of time, the fluid simply moved back into the arm. A more effective new approach to managing severe swelling is called CDP—for complete decongestive physiotherapy. This process involves sequential massage by a trained physical therapist, to work the fluid out of the arm. One excellent program called Lerner Lymphedema Services has centers in New York City, New Brunswick, New Jersey, Fort Lauderdale, Florida, and Boston, Massachusetts. It involves a monthlong program of massage, exercises, and compression bandaging. Patients are trained to do the massage, exercise, and bandaging themselves at home after the program is complete. Proper massage can make a big difference in the control of lymphedema. Unfortunately, it can be very costly and may not be covered by health insurance. However, I have written letters to insurance companies to pressure them to support my patients, and after being challenged on appeal, Medicare and other insurance groups have in fact come through and reimbursed women for this needed procedure. So it's worth a fight.

◆ WHAT CAN I DO ABOUT THE SORENESS AND NUMBNESS I FEEL SINCE LYMPH NODE REMOVAL?

About 70 percent of women who undergo lymph node surgery experience some soreness, numbness, and/or a sense of pulling or tightness in the breast and arm area afterward. Half of those who undergo lymph node surgery report postoperative tingling, stiffness, and pain. It's very important to be aware that this is normal and is not a sign of a breast cancer recurrence or a problem with the surgery itself. Usually, these

Pray for enough numbness to cancel out the soreness.

odd sensations recede—either through time alone, or with a change of position or short-term pain medication. Discuss your degree of discomfort with your doctor, so together you can map out an appropriate way to manage your problem. I have found, with my own patients, that just knowing that these feelings are normal goes a long way to making women feel better. The fear that something serious is going on is often more debilitating than the mild tingling or stiffness itself. And hopefully, with the advent of the far less invasive sentinel node biopsy (discussed on pages 176–79), these uncomfortable feelings will be eliminated.

◆ MY TREATMENT IS FINALLY COMPLETE AND I'M STARTING MY "LIFE AFTER CANCER." SHOULD I EAT ANY SPECIAL DIET?

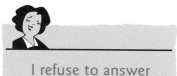

I refuse to answer any question with the word "diet" in it.

Not right away. I always advise my patients to take their time about making radical changes in their lifestyle after breast cancer. This has been an enormously stressful time—the last thing you need now is an additional stressor such as a wholesale change in your diet, eliminating alcohol, and so on. Believe it or not, I even tell smokers not to try to quit cold-turkey at this time, for two main reasons: first, quitting this way takes a huge psychological and physical toll, and second, it's not likely to last if you take it on at this vulnerable time. Your goal, certainly, should be to live as healthful a life as possible. There is evidence (discussed more fully on pages 91–93) that a low-fat, high-fiber diet may help lower your risk of breast cancer recurrence and of other cancers and other major diseases as well. So over time, with the help of a trained nutritionist, it's a great idea to improve your diet. The last thing anyone needs is excessive alcohol, so if you're a regular drinker, you should consider tapering off significantly—with time. But the bottom line, in the short term, is you should not make dramatic shifts in your behavior right away. If you love steak, don't renounce it the day your diagnosis comes in, or the day treatment ends. Don't eat it every night, either. Take a deep breath, set healthy priorities—e.g., quit smoking first, lower alcohol intake next, lower fat intake next—over the next several weeks or months. Your doctor should be able to help guide you in choosing the best changes to make first, and in how to time the design of your new lifestyle. Remember, too, that while your hope is to avoid a breast cancer recurrence, these kinds of lifestyle changes will go much further than that. A healthier lifestyle will make you feel and look better, and avoid countless life-threatening diseases that affect women of all ages. You deserve to live long and well after this ordeal of breast cancer is over.

I JUST FINISHED CHEMOTHERAPY. HOW CAN I REGAIN MY STRENGTH?

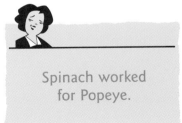

Spinach worked for Popeye.

One of the most common and intense side effects of chemotherapy is fatigue. In one study, 7 out of 10 women experienced profound tiredness as a result of chemotherapy. In addition to the direct toxic effects of the drugs, exhaustion can be caused by trouble sleeping, anxiety, and depression that can accompany breast cancer treatment.

The great news is, the vast majority of women regain their strength quite rapidly after chemotherapy is stopped. In general, 80 percent of your pretreatment strength returns within three months after chemotherapy, and 100 percent within a year. There are a few things you can do to help the process along, however. Eat a well-balanced, healthy diet (this is no time for food fads); establish a good, consistent sleeping pattern; and gradually return to an enjoyable exercise program. These three steps will help you to rebuild your strength and energy even as your body naturally heals itself. *Gradual* is the operative word, however: do *not* try to be superwoman immediately after stopping treatment. Let your body strengthen at its own natural pace.

Also keep in mind that depression (which is very common and normal after all treatments for breast cancer) can promote fatigue. Eating well, getting sleep, and exercising do help with depression, but many women find that some short-term counseling is also needed to help get over the difficult posttreatment hump. Support groups can be very useful at this time as well, as it is helpful to talk to other women experiencing the same sense of being "down" after the aggressive fight against cancer has moved into a different phase—that is, the long-awaited "life after cancer" phase. (See pages 229–31 for a more detailed discussion of support groups.)

◆ HOW CAN I CARE FOR MY SKIN DURING AND AFTER RADIATION THERAPY?

These days, "megavoltage" radiation therapy machines are widely available. This type of radiation beam spares the skin damage that was much more common in years past. Despite this advance, however, many women do have some skin effects from radiation therapy. The most common changes include some degree of redness, irritation, and peeling of the skin, not unlike the effect of a sunburn. The degree and type of skin irritation depends on the type of skin you have to begin with—some women will develop more reddish or pinkish skin, others more brownish skin. It is quite uncommon to develop severe breaks in the surface of the skin, but this does rarely occur. In general, women who receive *only* radiation therapy have fewer skin effects than women who receive *both* radiation therapy and chemotherapy at the same time. For this reason, when there is a choice (and there often is), we try to give these treatments in sequence rather than at the same time.

There are a few things you can do to lessen skin problems associated with radiation therapy. First, avoid any irritants to the skin:

◆ ◆ ◆ ◆ ◆ ◆ ◆ ◆ ◆ ◆ ◆ ◆ ◆ ◆ ◆ ◆ ◆ ◆ ◆ ◆

• Don't use perfume, cologne, or other perfumed products like antiperspirants during the several weeks of radiation therapy.

• Don't dye your hair, as peroxide and other such products can trickle onto your skin and further irritate it.

• Avoid tight clothing and underwire bras: if possible, this is a good time to use a cotton tank top under your clothing as an alternative. For women with very large breasts, this may not be practical, however. Choose loose, cotton clothing rather than restrictive and potentially irritating synthetics.

• Finally, try using some form of water-based lubricant on your skin after your treatments. You can use pure aloe gel, aquaphor, biophine (available widely in Europe and recently appearing in the U.S. as well), or vitamin A and D (A and D ointment) and combination creams. These creams can make a big difference in reducing irritation, dryness, and sensitivity caused by radiation therapy.

You can take solace in the fact that radiation-induced skin changes heal within several weeks of treatment. This is a temporary bother, rather than a long-term health complication.

◆ **WHAT IMMEDIATE TESTS SHOULD BE DONE AFTER MY TREATMENT FOR BREAST CANCER IS FINISHED?**

If you had surgery to remove calcifications that were malignant,
you should have a mammogram
before starting radiation therapy,
to be sure that the microcalcifications were completely removed.
This, unfortunately, is something
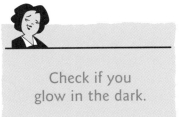

Check if you
glow in the dark.

that many people forget to do. Then, about six months after ra-
diation therapy is complete, do another mammogram on that breast, to make sure once again that no worrisome microcalcifications remain. Finally, be sure to have mammograms of both breasts on a yearly basis thereafter—and more frequently, at

your doctor's discretion, during the first year after surgery. (You do *not* need mammograms for breasts that were reconstructed after mastectomy.)

Sometimes, the type of treatment your doctor is planning to use will affect the type of tests you need. For example, if your doctor plans to use the chemotherapy drug Adriamycin (which can affect heart function), a test called a MUGA scan may be done to check your heart function before treatment is started.

Depending on the extent of your disease (which you will learn from the staging report that comes back after your surgery is done), your doctor may do additional tests to see if the cancer has spread to other parts of your body. For instance, you may need a CAT scan or a bone scan. These are not done routinely for every woman, but rather depend on the stage of your cancer. Abnormal blood tests (i.e., liver function tests) may also lead to further evaluation.

◆ MY CHEMOTHERAPY BROUGHT ON A SUDDEN AND SEVERE MENOPAUSE. WHAT CAN I DO NOW TO ALLEVIATE THESE TERRIBLE HOT FLASHES AND OTHER SYMPTOMS?

Menopause can be an uncomfortable time for many women, but for those who experience it suddenly, the sensations are often worse. Hot flashes can be especially severe; vaginal dryness and pain acute; sleep disturbance and mood changes more pronounced. Hot flashes can last for several years, although some women get over them in a matter of months. There are many treatments, both lifestyle changes and medications, that can lessen these symptoms. Unfortunately, one of the best treatments out there for menopausal discomfort—that is, hormone replacement therapy—is usually *not* given to women with breast cancer, since it is unknown whether estrogen causes an increased risk of cancer recurrence.

Other medications and vitamins that are often prescribed to help lessen the effects of hot flashes include:

• Megace, or megestrol acetate (20 mg, twice a day), is a progestin. This treatment was shown to reduce the frequency of hot flashes in a well-controlled study, with only one side effect: withdrawal menstrual bleeding one to two weeks after treatment was stopped. Megace is also an appetite enhancer and can promote weight gain. It has not been specifically studied in women who have had breast cancer or who are on tamoxifen.

• Clonidine (0.1 mg twice a day) was found to reduce both the frequency and severity of hot flashes, but had side effects such as dry mouth and constipation. Do not use clonidine if you have kidney problems.

• 800 IUs oral vitamin E per day; it's controversial whether this treatment makes a meaningful difference, but even if it does work, it may take a few weeks before you feel the effects of this treatment. The treatment is not toxic and has other health benefits, so it's worth a try.

• A combination of belladonna, phenobarbital, and ergotamine, which is often prescribed to fight hot flashes, actually does *not* help most women with either the frequency or the severity of hot flashes, can be habit-forming, and comes with a whole host of unpleasant side effects. It should not be taken by anyone with heart disease or impaired liver or kidney function.

• Antidepressants such as Effexor have been used with varying degrees of success. Talk to your doctor about this possible option.

• Benzodiazepan (i.e., Valium) at night may help, but can be habit-forming—talk to your doctor.

◆ ARE THERE NONDRUG APPROACHES TO LESSENING HOT FLASHES?

Yes. But first, avoid the many triggers to hot flashes, such as spicy foods, hot foods or beverages, alcohol, caffeine, and overly warm rooms. Dress in layers and be ready to strip down if a flash occurs. This

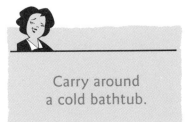

Carry around
a cold bathtub.

can be especially important at night, when hot flashes can disturb sleep. Try to sleep in a cool room, if possible, and keep ice water by the bed. While myth has it that menopause causes irritability, many researchers believe that it's the lack of sleep brought on by hot flashes, and not menopause itself, that causes such mood disturbance. Stress is another hot flash trigger—it's hard to stay clear of in this day and age, but do so whenever possible. Stress management techniques like deep breathing, meditation, massage, yoga, or even a long bubble bath can help reduce anxiety and in turn cut the number of hot flashes. Acupuncture also has been shown (anecdotally) to help.

Some recommend eating a diet rich in soy foods to alleviate menopausal hot flashes. This advice stems from the fact that women in rural Japan, whose diets are rich in soy-based foods, tend to have far fewer hot flashes than do American women. The theory is that these foods are rich in plant estrogens, which may do some of the good work of estrogen (fighting menopausal symptoms) but not the bad (fueling breast cancer). Soy-based foods, such as soy flour, whole soybeans, soy protein, soy milk, tofu, miso, and tempeh have plenty of "isoflavones," which are a class of plant estrogens. But in soy isolates and concentrate, such as some processed foods, the amount of soy varies—for example, soy sauce made from hydrolyzed vegetable protein has *none!* We know that the most potent soy extract is mega soy extract—it contains almost 40 percent of pure soy isoflavones. But here's the catch: We don't know if women with estrogen receptor–positive breast tumors should use soy. In addition, the relationship between soy and tamoxifen has not been fully explored. We just don't know whether women who get lots of plant estrogen in the form of foods are at risk for fueling existing (or new) breast tumors. In general, we believe that the best type of soy to use is "soy genistein," which inhibits the growth of cells and new blood vessels and fights the growth of some estrogen receptor–positive tumors. Dry roasted soybeans are an excellent source of genistein. But talk to your doctor about the use of soy, and remember that moderation, and not gorging, is key.

Another plant estrogen that gets a lot of attention in the fight against hot flashes is black cohosh. It has not been rigorously studied, and can theoretically produce risk associated with estrogen. Talk to your doctor before using it or any other herbal remedy for menopausal symptoms.

How can I manage the vaginal dryness and discomfort that resulted from my "chemotherapy menopause"?

Vaginal dryness and discomfort is a common symptom of menopause, and can be more pronounced in women who undergo menopause suddenly—as in the case of some women who receive chemotherapy. The discomfort can be so severe as to make sexual intercourse terribly painful or outright impossible. Also common are chronic itching or irritation of the vulva (the outside of the vagina), the sense that you have to urinate when you really don't, and some leakage of urine during coughs or sneezes. Be sure that your doctor rules out the many different health problems—apart from menopausal change—that could be causing your symptoms, such as vaginal infection of some type, a urinary tract infection, allergy to a chemical in a product you're using or the material in your undergarments, and so on. Once it has been clearly established that a lack of estrogen due to sudden menopause is the culprit, you can start to take action.

First, a diet rich in the plant estrogens (like soy) discussed earlier may help some women. (Always talk to your doctor about the potential risks of estrogen-based plants and herbs, however, in your case.) But often, a much more direct solution is needed—such as a water-based vaginal moisturizer like Astroglide, Replens, Slip, and K-Y Long-Lasting Vaginal Moisturizer. But some women find them too goopy and messy for regular use. As a group, though, these water-based lubricants are less sloppy and irritating than oil-based products like Vaseline and baby oil. (And don't forget, oil-based lubricants can erode the material in condoms and diaphragms, while water-based ones pose no harm to these contraceptives. If you're thinking "why would I use a condom when I'm already past menopause," think again: you're still potentially at risk for sexually transmitted diseases, so condoms can be lifesaving even if you don't need them to prevent pregnancy.)

Don't forget the old standby, saliva (your own or your partner's)—it's a helpful lubricant for many women. Of course, if there's any infection present in the mouth, like oral herpes sores, there is still a risk of passing it to the genital area—so use common sense.

Having sex, as uncomfortable as it may be, is another solution for vaginal dryness and atrophy. Intercourse helps keep the vagina healthy and flexible. But because vaginal discomfort often makes women avoid sex altogether, a vicious cycle can be set up: Vaginal discomfort leads to no sex, which leads to further vaginal discomfort. You need to have a patient and cooperative sexual partner to make postmenopausal sex comfortable. Working together to find the right lubricant(s), taking time during foreplay, and having sex as regularly as possible will all help.

Finally, the best treatment for vaginal dryness, irritation, and atrophy is estrogen cream—which can be used as a topical cream or in the form of Estring, a vaginal ring. The trouble is, even though this cream is placed on the skin of the vagina, some of it does in fact get absorbed into the bloodstream, which could pose a risk to women with estrogen receptor–positive breast tumors. You can be sure not much estrogen gets into the bloodstream, however, because estrogen cream has little or no effect on such systemic problems as hot flashes and bone loss associated with menopause. I tend to recommend estrogen cream only for that woman after breast cancer whose quality of life is so severely damaged by vaginal dryness that she finds herself miserable as a result—for instance, a woman who absolutely cannot have intercourse, or who has chronic vaginal discomfort. If you feel this way, then certainly discuss the use of vaginal estrogen cream ring with your doctor.

◆ How can i protect my bones after a sudden chemotherapy-induced menopause?

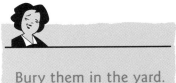

Bone loss, or osteoporosis, is one of the most serious complications of menopause. Tens of thousands of women fracture bones every year as a result of this debilitating problem. We've spent so much time talking about the adverse effects of estrogen

Bury them in the yard. It works for my dog.

in regard to breast cancer risk, it's easy to forget that estrogen plays some important and lifesaving roles in the female body as well. And preserving bone integrity is one of estrogen's "good" jobs. When estrogen is lost with a sudden menopause, the bones can thin rapidly, becoming more porous and brittle as well. Again, hormone replacement therapy is one of the best treatments—but it is often not recommended for women with breast cancer. So it's important to look at other ways to protect your bones.

First, turn to diet and exercise. Calcium is the dietary building block of bone, and most American women get too little of it each day. Postmenopausal women who are not taking hormone replacement should consume 1500 mg of calcium per day in divided doses—yet most get a quarter of this amount at best. Talk to your doctor about the right amount for you, given your sudden menopause and the effect this can have on your bones.

It's not easy to get 1500 mg of calcium per day. To give you an idea of why, consider this: an 8-ounce glass of milk has about 300 mg; an ounce of cheddar cheese has about 200 mg; a 3-ounce serving salmon with bones in it has about 167 mg; 8 ounces of yogurt has about 450 mg; and a cup of broccoli has about 136 mg. Calcium-fortified orange juice is a good source, with 350 mg per cup.

Many women who drink coffee with milk in it think they're getting their daily needed calcium. Not only are they not coming close to their daily recommended requirement, but they're also making a big mistake: the caffeine in coffee counteracts the effects of the calcium, causing you to excrete it rather than absorb it. The same is true of excessive protein and sodium in the diet. Eating too much fat will interfere with calcium absorption.

Do be sure to get some vitamin D in your diet (800 IU is recommended), as it promotes calcium absorption and helps your bones to use that calcium. If you drink vitamin D–fortified milk or eat vitamin D–fortified cereals, you're probably getting enough. Also, exposure to sunlight in moderate amounts allows your body to synthesize vitamin D in your own skin.

Finally, if you just can't eat or drink all that calcium, talk to your doctor about whether a daily calcium supplement would be right for you.

◆ WHAT ABOUT EXERCISE FOR MY BONES?

Weight-bearing exercise helps promote bone density. So any exercise in which you carry your own body weight is a good choice: walking, jogging, dancing, playing tennis, weight training, and so on. If you've had a surgical biopsy or lumpectomy, wait about two weeks before resuming your exercise regimen (and always check with your own doctor first). Also be sure to support your breasts with a good, comfortable sports bra. If you had nodes removed or breast reconstruction, wait until your drain is removed to start exercising (and ask your plastic surgeon to discuss your exercise regimen with your breast doctor).

Try to do as much weight-bearing exercise as possible without hurting your joints (walking, for example, is a lot easier on the joints than jogging, and just as good for the bones). Shoot for a half-hour of weight-bearing exercise several times per week. And increase the amount of general weight-bearing exercise you do during normal everyday activities, such as walking up and down stairs instead of taking the elevator, walking to work instead of taking the bus, and so on.

◆ ◆

Swimming, while a wonderful exercise for other reasons, is not a weight-bearing exercise and therefore does not offer much protection to the bones. It is great for increasing range of motion after breast cancer surgery, however.

LONG-TERM AFTERCARE:

WENDIE JO SPERBER

What cancer did was teach me about people, and teach me about myself. For one, it made me realize that I seriously had to start taking care of myself, which was very hard for someone like me, whose drug of choice has always been sugar. But the most important lesson I learned had nothing to do with food, and really had nothing to do with cancer! What I learned most was the importance of being okay with me, about loving and believing in myself. The cancer was kind of a wake-up call. It forced me to look at what was going on, what the lessons were in my life at the time.

◆ **I WAS DIAGNOSED AND TREATED FOR BREAST CANCER OVER A YEAR AGO, BUT I'M STILL SCARED OF A RECURRENCE. IS THIS NORMAL?**

There is enormous variability in the degree of fear women experience after breast cancer. Some women suffer from nightmares, don't want to touch their bodies at all—especially their surgical scars—and even dress in the dark. Others make a rapid emotional recovery, thrilled to be alive and ready to move on. I always tell my patients that it's important to have a chance to mourn after breast cancer. The mourning or grieving process is for the breast cancer experience itself, and for the loss of a breast—or even part of a breast. Many people are understanding about the deep sense of loss after mastectomy, but women who go through lumpectomy—removal of the tumor, not the entire breast—often do not get their fair share of compassion from loved ones. They're often told how lucky they are that they didn't have to lose their breast—rather than consoled for how painful the breast cancer experience must have been. As a result of this lack of concern, I've seen many women become depressed after lumpectomy. The grieving or mourning process is important for some women regardless of the degree of change in their bodies—regardless of the extent of the cancer, the extent of the treatment, and their physical reaction to the treatment.

◆ DO YOU HAVE SUGGESTIONS ABOUT HOW TO SHORTEN THE PERIOD OF GRIEVING AND FEARING?

If you find that your terror about a recurrence, or your anger and pain about your changed body is just too hard to resolve on your own, seek the right kind of counseling. Signs that your emotional health needs tending include chronic lack of

Do it in February; it's a shorter month.

sleep (or excessive sleep), a lack of interest in or energy for normal everyday activities and relationships, a lack of interest in sex, inability to concentrate on normal responsibilities or inability to do your job, or a marked change in appetite. Many different kinds of health practitioners can help you make your way back to your old self, including psychiatrists, psychologists, social workers, members of the clergy, or other breast cancer survivors—sometimes in support group settings. (I'll talk more about support groups in a moment.) There is also a relatively new and growing group of subspecialists, called psychooncologists—these doctors are especially attuned to the emotional issues related to cancer treatment and recovery.

Thankfully, now that breast cancer is a much more open topic and women are sharing their feelings and experiences more than ever before, there is a great deal of help out there. You do not need to endure the emotional trauma of this disease alone, any more than you did the physical trauma. Sometimes, talk therapy is the solution; in other cases, some kind of additional physical treatment needs to be done to help restore your confidence and pleasure in your own body. For instance, some women who opted not to have breast reconstruction after mastectomy may find that they need to return for this procedure in order to feel "whole" once again. Others may be dissatisfied with their surgical result and want further corrective surgery, if possible, to improve the cosmetic result. Every case is different. But in my experience, the vast majority are solvable, given the right kind of support. Ask your doctor or nurse to refer you to an appropriate support group or service for your need.

◆ I'M WORRIED THAT MY SEX LIFE WON'T RETURN TO NORMAL AFTER MY BREAST SURGERY. ANY ADVICE?

Most women in good sexual relationships *before* breast cancer find themselves in good sexual relationships afterward. Of course, this requires some time—for most women, the last thing on their minds during the treatment phase

> Screw your brains out before the operation.

of breast cancer is having sex. Treatments can be tiring—both emotionally and physically draining. But afterward, given a loving and supportive partner, sex usually survives breast cancer. I find that the best cases are those in which the partner goes through the entire diagnostic and treatment process, and therefore knows what to expect—both physically, and emotionally—after breast cancer. In these cases, the scars are not surprising or scary; the fears are understandable; and the recovery process becomes a joint affair.

That said, of course there are exceptions. Women who have no sexual partner—or soul mate, for that matter—*before* breast cancer may have a harder time developing a normal sex life *afterward*. There are fears about dating someone new and exposing the private changes your body has been through. Or, for those in unstable relationships that are lacking in emotional support, sometimes the partner's reaction to a major physical change is a big disappointment. Some women face rejection when they come home with both a changed physique *and* psyche. Sometimes, these problems are not solvable—and you may discover that you're with the wrong person. Certainly the last thing you want to do is stay in a destructive relationship that hammers in the negatives about your body rather than celebrating the positives. In other cases, couples counseling and some education for your partner about what has actually changed—and what has remained the same—about your body after breast cancer can make a big, positive difference.

Remember, too, that for some women, there are good physical explanations for sexual problems after breast cancer. Take, for example, women who go through an early and sudden menopause as a result of chemotherapy (this is discussed in greater detail on pages 213–14). These women experience vaginal dryness and pain which can make sexual intercourse difficult or impossible. There are several solutions for this type of discomfort (see pages 216–19 in this chapter). Whatever you do, don't let these physical impediments to sexual enjoyment go untreated. Your sex life is an integral part of your return to loving your body and getting over the physical shock of breast cancer. Most important, don't fear talking openly to your doctor about these issues. You're not going to raise any issue he or she hasn't heard before. And if you don't speak up, you'll never find the help you deserve.

Keep one final thing in mind: The more comfortable you are with your own body after breast cancer treatment, the more likely your partner will mirror your views. The sooner you come to terms with life after breast cancer, and learn to love and trust your body again, the sooner your sexual partner will pick up on that comfort and relax as well.

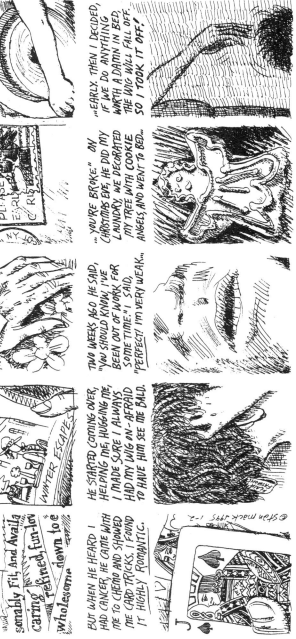
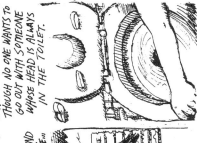
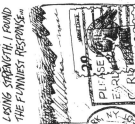
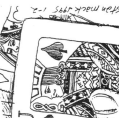

(Courtesy of Stan Mack)

◆ **My husband treats me with kid gloves ever since my breast cancer surgery. I know he means well, but I want to move past this artificial stage. What can I do?**

The best way to get partners over the worrying phase is to include them every step of the way. Have them present during any discussions with your doctor about your life after breast cancer—such as what exercises you can and should do, and what you should expect from your body. If you weren't a tennis ace before breast cancer surgery, you aren't likely to be one afterward. But you can, and *should*, expect to be as normal, strong, and effective after healing from breast cancer surgery as you were before you were ever diagnosed. You are not an invalid, you are not weak, you are not frail. But without proper education, your partner has no way of knowing this. I've had spouses, partners, and children come into the office to discuss all aspects of treatment and recovery, just to set the record straight. And there are support groups for family members, including children, as well (see page 278 for details on finding such a group). Yes, women do experience twinges in the arm after having lymph nodes removed, for example. But when partners learn about these sensations and come to know what's normal and expected, they will lose their worries and inhibitions faster and help you move back to the normalcy you're craving.

◆ **It has been many years since my treatment for breast cancer and my doctor considers me cured. But I still suffer from nightmares about the disease. Will this ever stop?**

What you experience isn't unheard of. I had a patient recently who was eighteen years past her breast cancer diagnosis, and who is still "scared to death." While time generally lessens the fear, there are a few reasons why the passing of the years can have a different—and more negative—effect. For one thing, as you grow older and have more aches and pains and health problems in general, you become more fearful about your overall health. This can trigger new concerns about breast cancer—either a recurrence, or a new breast cancer. For other women, there are more regular reminders—for instance, the yearly mammogram—that allow fear to rear its ugly head again and again. You may never totally eradicate your fears. However, there are ways to lessen them. In addition to the counseling discussed earlier in this chapter, there are simple changes in your behavior that can lessen occasional fear. For instance, go to the movies or out with a friend the night before your mammogram rather than sitting home mulling over your worries. And make yourself as busy as possible before the test itself—distraction is a good weapon against fear.

◆ I WORRY ABOUT EVERY LUMP AND BUMP IN MY BODY NOW. WHERE DOES BREAST CANCER ACTUALLY SPREAD, AND WHAT ARE THE SIGNS OF A RECURRENCE?

There are different kinds of breast cancer recurrences, including *local* (in or under the skin of the chest wall, in or near the surgical scar); *regional* (in the lymph nodes under the arm); and *distant* (in other parts of the body, such as the bones, lungs, and brain). Most recurrences appear within five years of a mastectomy; however, recurrences can appear after fifteen to twenty years, particularly after lumpectomy. In general, having a recurrence after five years means a better prognosis than having a recurrence in the first two years.

As for the signs to look for, they vary. Many people are unaware that it's possible to have a recurrence after mastectomy. They figure that if the breast is gone, you can't have any more breast cancer. I wish that were true, but it isn't. After a mastectomy, a local recurrence might show up as a lump or nodule on the chest wall under the mastectomy scar—sometimes it's visible, sometimes it can be felt under the skin. A recurrence in the lymph nodes under the armpit might appear as a lump as well.

A recurrence after lumpectomy can occur at the site of the surgical scar, or a little farther away. Or, you can get a cancer in a totally different site—in which case there may be some uncertainty as to whether this is a recurrence or a new cancer. It's extremely important to continue to have mammograms after lumpectomy, as a third to a half of recurrences after lumpectomy and radiation therapy are detected solely by follow-up mammograms. When there is a great deal of scarring, or thickening of the breast skin, radiologists sometimes use a special radio-opaque wire at the site of the lumpectomy scar to show the lumpectomy site more clearly on the mammogram. This helps in the detection of cancers that may be "hiding" near lots of scar tissue. Other recurrences after lumpectomy are found on physical examinations of the breast—so it's also critical to see your doctor regularly for follow-up breast exams.

The symptoms of more distant recurrences depend largely on where the cancer has spread. Spread to the bone can cause bone pain, or trouble walking; spread to the lungs can produce trouble breathing, shortness of breath, or a dry cough; spread to the brain can cause difficulty with balance, headaches, and visual problems; spread to the spine can cause back pain or leg weakness; spread to the liver can show up on an abnormal blood test. But you mustn't make yourself crazy thinking that every pain or problem is a cancer recurrence. During your routine follow-up appointments with your oncologist, you will be monitored for any signs of recurrence. Certainly you should tell your doctor about any new or unusual pains or problems that you haven't experienced before. But try to remind yourself that your body experienced its ups and downs before you were ever diagnosed with breast cancer.

◆ ◆ ◆ ◆ ◆ ◆ ◆ ◆ ◆ ◆ ◆ ◆ ◆ ◆ ◆ ◆ ◆ ◆ ◆ ◆

> The American Society of Clinical Oncologists (ASCO) recommends that all women who have had breast cancer have a careful history and physical exam every three to six months for the first three years after primary therapy; every six to twelve months for the next two years; and then annually thereafter.

◆ I KEEP READING HOW IMPORTANT IT IS TO COMMUNICATE WITH MY DOCTOR, WITH A GIVE-AND-TAKE. WHAT CAN I EXPECT MY DOCTOR TO TALK ABOUT, AND WHAT TOPICS SHOULD I RAISE MYSELF?

Of course this depends a lot on the type of person your doctor is, but there are a few generalizations to keep in mind. Doctors are most likely to talk about the *physical* aspects of breast cancer recovery—that is, what to do with your drains after surgery; how to help your skin recover after radiation therapy; what kinds of follow-up tests you will need; when to return to the doctor's office; and perhaps how to massage and lessen your surgical scars. This is the arena in which most doctors feel comfortable—your physical recovery and survival.

Beyond these topics, there are many important issues related to your treatment and ongoing quality of life that your doctor is less likely to discuss. These include such subjects as your emotional health after breast cancer; your sexual relationships; the symptoms of sudden menopause; and the use of complementary, non-mainstream therapies. Now the fact that your doctor doesn't raise these subjects may not mean that he or she lacks information on them. Sometimes, it's a matter of you taking the lead and asking questions straight-out. In other cases, though, your doctor may really be lacking in information on these matters. This is why I have tried to dedicate a good number of pages of this book to the non-physical questions so many women have—and why the Resources section at the end of this book is chock-full of places where you can go to get additional support for these kinds of problems and questions.

◆ WHAT'S THE VALUE OF LONG-TERM SUPPORT GROUPS?

Support groups serve different purposes at different times. Immediately after diagnosis and during treatment, they can be important not only for emotional support but also as a source of vital information about treatment options, side ef-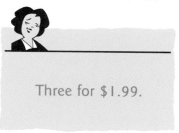fects to treatment, and many other pressing concerns. These early support groups usually run for about eight sessions or so.

Three for $1.99.

Later, though, after treatment is complete, support groups can play a quite different role. I have seen women in good, strong support groups develop powerful long-term bonds—friendships in a formalized setting that make the road to full emotional and physical recovery easier to manage. In some cases, other family members also reap the benefits of these long-term support groups. For example, I know of one husband who lost his wife to breast cancer, and decided to join her support group to help him through the pain of his loss, and to make him feel more connected to the world in which she had lived. The women who gave his wife the support she needed are now giving a needed boost to him. I am always amazed and impressed at the power of support groups to heal patients in ways that we doctors cannot.

◆ I'M NOT A BIG "GROUP" PERSON. ARE THERE OTHER OPTIONS FOR MORE PRIVATE FORMS OF SUPPORT?

Yes—in fact, one of the most successful approaches to support that I have used in my own practice is the "buddy system," in which I match one patient with another who has a similar stage of disease as well as a similar life background. These "buddies" can go through chemotherapy together; or they can simply talk on the phone occasionally to share experiences, fears, or success stories. Sometimes, all a woman wants is to see a buddy's surgical scar or reconstruction result. Buddies can serve many different purposes. Ask your doctor or nursing staff if they can recommend a buddy for you.

Also, the "self-help" model of recovery, founded by the New York–based group SHARE (Self-help for Women with Breast and Ovarian Cancer) and available in different forms around the country, offers a number of educational seminars and programs through which you can help heal yourself. For example, taking classes in yoga, relaxation, meditation, visualization, and other means of stress reduction can help you relieve your emotional and physical stress in the privacy of your own home, any time of day.

WHO SHOULD LEAD AN EFFECTIVE SUPPORT GROUP, AND WHO SHOULD BE INCLUDED?

The people who run support groups are formally called "facilitators." The name shows you what their main role should be—that is, a supportive guide who enables fruitful discussions to take place among the group members. Support groups are not lectures, but rather they are give-and-take sessions where women share both their fears and their successes, their questions and their knowledge about the breast cancer experience. The best support groups are made up of women with similar prognoses and who are on similar life "wavelengths"—for example, women with young children, older women with grown children, divorced women, single women, and so on. The greater the similarities in life experience, the greater the value of each woman's input will be for the group as a whole. You can imagine that if you're seventy-five and living with a retired spouse, your issues about dealing with breast cancer will be different from those of a thirty-year-old woman with two young kids. Or, if you're in a long-term, stable sexual relationship, your issues will differ from a woman who is single and dating after breast cancer. Or if your prognosis is excellent, you may not want to be in a group with women whose prognoses are more guarded.

As far as who makes the best facilitator for a breast cancer support group—well, that depends. Support groups can be run by breast cancer survivors with no other health care background; they can be run by psychiatrists, psychologists, social workers, and others in the mental health care field. In my experience, properly trained breast cancer survivors often make the best facilitators. These take on the feeling of self-help groups, and can be enormously empowering for all women involved. It is very important, though, that any potential facilitator has been properly screened and trained as an appropriate group leader. The last thing anyone wants is to end up in a group led by an emotionally unsettled survivor. The American Cancer Society has a useful list of questions to ask in training programs for support group facilitators, including: "Is she well-adjusted and emotionally stable?"; "Does she have a knowledge of professional ethics?"; and "Will she maintain confidentiality?" I personally recommend that she be at least two years out of her own treatment regimen as well.

◆ SHOULD I BE WORRIED ABOUT WEIGHT GAIN AFTER BREAST CANCER TREATMENT?

There is some evidence that weight gain, common after chemotherapy, can increase the risk of breast cancer recurrence in postmenopausal women. The theory holds that excessive weight—especially in the belly area—increases the levels of unhealthy estrogen in the body, thereby fueling some kinds of breast cancer. Also, excessive fat increases the production of insulin growth factor in the body, another substance that can promote tumor growth. There also may be increased contaminants in animal fats that are foreign or xenoestrogens. These issues are currently being studied by researchers, so at this point there are no black-and-white answers. However, I always tell my patients that it stands to reason that the more fit you are, the better you will fight breast cancer and other diseases as well. Making the smart lifestyle changes discussed throughout this book—e.g., lowering fat intake, increasing fiber intake, stopping smoking, and reducing alcohol intake—can only help, and certainly won't hurt. Less fat on your body means a lower risk of a great number of life-threatening illnesses, and also improves your mobility and overall quality of life. Talk to your doctor about choosing an ideal weight for your body type and then set a realistic plan for reaching that goal over a sensible period of time. Crash diets are not recommended now, in the aftermath of breast cancer treatment—or at any time of life, for that matter.

◆ I'VE HEARD THAT AIR TRAVEL IS NOT RECOMMENDED AFTER BREAST CANCER SURGERY. IS THIS TRUE?

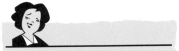

There is some evidence—albeit unscientific evidence—that *prolonged* (e.g., international or cross-country) air travel can promote swelling in the arm after lymph node removal. I discussed lymphedema, or fluid retention in the arm, earlier in this chapter (see pages 196–208). It is

Actually, air travel is not recommended *during* breast cancer surgery.

possible that the pressure of *prolonged* air travel would exacerbate this problem. For this reason, I suggest that air travelers who have had underarm lymph nodes removed use a compression sleeve during travel, to help force fluid out of the arm. If you don't already have such a sleeve, talk to your doctor about obtaining one—and having it custom fit—before your trip. Also try to keep your arm elevated during flight.

◆ ARE THERE SPECIALTY STORES THAT CATER TO WOMEN'S NEEDS AFTER CANCER?

Yes, and they are becoming more and more common. One woman, Linda Secher, who used to work for the American Cancer Society "Look Good . . . Feel Better" program, has launched nine such boutiques across the United States. These stores cater to the needs of women after treatment for breast cancer and other cancers. Because they work through a warehouse system, they are able to supply women all over the country. See page 276 in the Resources section for details on contacting these shops.

Products include such things as wigs, turbans, and hats to use if there is hair thinning or loss as a result of chemotherapy; prosthetic breasts for women who had mastectomies without breast reconstruction; compression sleeves to reduce the swelling of lymphedema; special aluminum-free deodorants that can safely be used during radiation therapy or during mammograms; special topical creams to be used after radiation therapy; and many other important products and garments.

ARE THESE DEVICES EXPENSIVE, AND DOES INSURANCE HELP PAY FOR THEM?

Sometimes. Usually, insurance covers part of the cost—check with your own insurer to find out exactly what, and how much, is covered. The same goes for Medicare and Medicaid— some things are covered, and others not. For example, Medicare covers prostheses and bras and sometimes covers wigs. Medicaid covers prostheses, bras, and wigs.

Unfortunately, these are expensive products. A synthetic wig can cost $200 or less, but a natural wig costs upwards of $2,000. Prostheses, which are made of silicone, cost anywhere from $60 to $400; customized versions can cost up to $3,000. (There's a new prosthesis on the market that sticks to the chest—so it doesn't slip around. But if you tend to perspire a lot, it won't stick—so this is not recommended for you.) Special bras cost about $18 to $60 and have a pocket to fit your prosthetic breast; your doctor should write you a prescription for lifetime use, which covers two bras every six months and one prosthesis. Lymphedema sleeves cost about $50 to $55, and you can buy a cotton *inner* sleeve to wear if you are allergic to the Lycra in the lymphedema sleeve itself.

◆ ◆

◆ How should I care for my prosthetic breast?

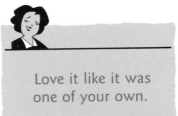

You should treat it as if it were real skin: wash it every day, dry it with a towel, keep it in its cradle to maintain its shape, avoid cats or other animals that might scratch or poke it, and avoid pins and needles (at the tailor, for example), which

> Love it like it was one of your own.

could puncture it. The bottom line—keep it as clean and safe from abuse as you would your own breast.

◆ Are there other cancer tests that I should have on a regular, ongoing basis?

The American Cancer Society recommends the following screening tests, at these recommended intervals.

THE PAP TEST FOR CANCER OF THE CERVIX: All women over the age of eighteen, or as soon as you become sexually active (whatever your age), should have this test *every year*. They add that women who have had three consecutive normal Pap smears, and who have *no* risk factors for cervical cancer, can be tested less often, at their doctors' discretion. The key risk factors for cervical cancer are (1) cigarette smoking; (2) having more than one sexual partner; and (3) having the viruses HPV (human papillomavirus) or HIV (the virus that causes AIDS). But I want to stress that because the Pap test is not always perfect (there are lab errors, recording errors, and other potential mishaps), your best defense is an annual Pap test regardless of your risk factor status.

A PELVIC EXAM BY YOUR DOCTOR: All women over the age of eighteen, or as soon as you become sexually active (whatever your age), *every year*.

COLON CANCER SCREENING: All women over the age of fifty should have a yearly fecal occult blood test (test for hidden blood in the stool) plus one of the following screening regimens:

> a flexible sigmoidoscopy and digital rectal exam every five years;
>
> or a colonoscopy and digital rectal exam every ten years;
>
> or a double-contrast barium enema and digital rectal exam every five to ten years.

However, if you have a family or personal history of colon/rectal cancer or polyps, your doctor may recommend more frequent screening. And some physicians recommend a yearly digital rectal exam (the physical exam by your doctor) every year for *all* patients, regardless of their history of disease.

The American Cancer Society also offers this extremely helpful anagram to help you watch for signs of cancer.

CAUTION:

C—a Change in bowel habits
A—A sore that won't go away
U—Unusual bleeding or discharge
T—Thick spot or lump in breast or anywhere else
I—Indigestion (bad, and more than occasional) and trouble swallowing
O—Obvious change in wart or mole
N—Nagging cough or unusually hoarse voice

Any of these signs should bring you to the doctor for a checkup. More often than not, they will prove harmless, but as you've learned, the earlier you catch cancer, the more treatable it is—so you can only help yourself by seeking medical attention swiftly.

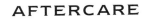

AFTERCARE

```
Y  E  A  P  C  Y  T  K  D  R  A  V  D  M  E  Y
E  X  E  O  D  O  A  B  O  D  Y  I  M  A  G  E
C  E  S  B  U  E  K  L  E  H  E  O  N  M  K  Y
N  R  U  Y  B  Z  I  D  G  E  F  Q  S  G  F  N
T  C  A  Q  U  J  N  A  Q  T  X  N  S  E  L  N
S  I  P  T  N  Q  G  N  W  S  K  A  I  M  I  J
E  S  O  E  Z  P  S  L  W  E  N  L  S  S  V  Q
X  E  N  H  Y  F  T  Z  V  V  E  D  I  S  I  I
W  E  E  Q  D  N  O  O  L  R  S  D  S  D  N  B
F  I  M  U  S  B  C  K  G  U  O  I  E  D  G  Y
L  P  G  P  F  B  K  G  T  Y  C  G  H  I  P  H
U  X  V  E  W  K  K  X  S  P  I  M  T  E  Q  F
R  B  D  C  G  Y  Y  F  U  G  X  F  S  T  K  E
K  J  H  V  Y  A  M  E  R  R  B  W  O  T  E  I
A  S  A  N  I  T  Y  O  T  H  C  N  R  N  P  H
E  E  A  G  D  Q  D  G  U  A  D  Y  P  A  U  I
```

Find and circle the following words:

BODY IMAGE	MENOPAUSE	SEX
DIET	PROSTHESIS	TAKING STOCK
EXERCISE	RELIEF	TRUST
LIVING	SANITY	WIG

7

BREAST CANCER:
The Future

FRAN VISCO, PRESIDENT,
NATIONAL BREAST CANCER COALITION

In 1987 when I was diagnosed with breast cancer, my options for treatment were virtually identical to those of a woman facing the same situation twenty years earlier. But today I see the beginnings of a new world and an entirely new and different future for women with breast cancer.

I am hopeful about a woman's future—a future where breast cancer is no longer part of our vocabulary. While we have had some success, we have a long way to go to achieve that goal. The leaps we have made in breast cancer research are due primarily to the efforts of women with breast cancer and the women and men concerned about this issue who have come together to demand an end to this disease.

With their help, we have been able to ensure necessary federal research funding, fight for access to quality health care for all women, and bring our voice—that of advocates—to every table where important decisions about women's health are made.

I look forward to the promise of a future in which scientists know what causes breast cancer, and doctors know how to cure it. A future in which respectful and effective health care is available to every woman, regardless of her ability to pay for it. A future in which we can throw away our buttons and banners, tell our activists to relax, dismantle our national network of advocates. A future in which we can gather for conversation and celebration instead of strategy sessions, because breast cancer has been eradicated.

◆ ◆ ◆ ◆ ◆ ◆ ◆ ◆ ◆ ◆ ◆ ◆ ◆ ◆ ◆ ◆ ◆ ◆ ◆

◆ IN GENERAL TERMS, WHERE IS THE MANAGEMENT OF
BREAST CANCER HEADED IN THE NEXT DECADE?

Naturally the long-term goal in the treatment of any disease, including breast cancer, is to cure or eradicate the illness altogether.
But to be perfectly honest, while I would love to be wrong and
wind up out of business, I don't see that happening in the next
ten years. What I do see, however, is extremely important and
positive. I believe that with the advent of new therapies, new diagnostic tools, and new ways of determining women at greatest
risk of getting breast cancer, we will soon be able to manage even
advanced breast cancer as a chronic illness—not unlike diabetes,
for example. What do I mean by this? I see a time in the very
near future in which even those women with relatively advanced
breast cancer will live long, productive lives with this disease in
check. They will die of old age, after waging a series of battles
with breast cancer from time to time over the years. The disease
will be fought back into remission repeatedly. If you were told
you had heart disease, or severe diabetes, you might expect to live
a long life dotted with drug treatments, and perhaps occasional
operations—but most of the time you would expect to lead an
active and rich life. The same will be true of even the toughest
cases of breast cancer. The fights won't necessarily be easy, and
they certainly aren't fun, but women will increasingly be the win-
ners. And there will be countless elderly grandmothers telling of
their battles with breast cancer.

◆ THE DISCOVERY OF THE GENES FOR BREAST CANCER
GOT SO MUCH PRESS AND GENERATED SO MUCH
EXCITEMENT. BUT HOW IMPORTANT WERE THESE
DISCOVERIES IN TERMS OF THE FUTURE FIGHT
AGAINST BREAST CANCER?

The discovery of mutations on the genes BRCA1 and BRCA2
were exciting and important, but in many ways represent just
the tip of the iceberg in terms of the future war against breast
cancer. Remember that these particular gene mutations account

for just 5–10 percent of all breast cancers. This is a critical beginning. But only a beginning. I envision a time within ten or twenty years when we will be able to hand every woman a literal map of her genetic makeup, and part of that map will include a whole host of genes, and genetic mutations, that boost the risk for various diseases—including breast cancer. Already researchers are looking at a variety of other so-called susceptibility genes for breast cancer. Each individual susceptibility gene may raise a woman's risk of getting breast cancer by just a tiny amount—but if you have lots of them put together, your risk multiplies. What kinds of genes am I talking about? Well, for example, there are several variations on enzymes or proteins created by our bodies that are responsible for the metabolism of the hormone estrogen. If, for example, we don't handle estrogen well—because of some genetic predisposition or some environmental exposure that triggers a genetic mistake—we may be at increased risk of breast cancer. Or perhaps it's an abnormality in the way we process fat in the body. Or how we react to nicotine. There are thought to be many of these subtle, hard-to-identify genetic abnormalities that work as a group to increase our overall risk of breast and other cancers. The greater our understanding of these many elusive genes, the greater will be our ability both to target treatments at these abnormalities and also to identify and protect women at greatest risk.

◆ WHAT DOES THE FUTURE HOLD IN TERMS OF OUR UNDERSTANDING OF HOW GENES INTERACT WITH THE ENVIRONMENT TO CAUSE BREAST CANCER?

It is becoming increasingly clear that genes may strongly predispose us to many diseases, including breast cancer, but that often some type of "cofactor" in the environment is also needed to trigger a given disease. Take the case of a breast cancer gene called the "ataxia telangiectasia gene"—which is carried by a staggering 2.6 million people in the U.S. It is known that for people who carry this particular gene, exposure to ionizing radiation (either through occupational hazards, or through diagnostic tests)

greatly increases the risk of breast cancer. In fact, it's possible that
women who carry this gene might be at increased risk of breast
cancer even as a result of the small radiation exposure from
screening mammography. (This dose of radiation is of *no* concern for other women.) Fortunately, this is an extremely rare cir-
cumstance, and I mention it as just one example of a situation in
which our ability to identify and understand a genetic predisposition can be combined with our knowledge of an environmental risk factor for cancer. Environmental exposures can also
change our genes. The more we discover, the better our chance
of targeting and protecting particular groups of women from
dangerous exposures.

◆ IF THERE WERE TO BE A "MAGIC BULLET" CURE FOR BREAST CANCER, WHAT WOULD YOU PREDICT IT TO BE?

One of the things we've come to understand about breast cancer, and other cancers for that matter, is that it is not one single
entity. There are many different types—determined by many
factors we've talked about throughout this book—that determine where the tumor starts, how aggressive it is, what kinds of
drugs and treatments it responds to, and so on. Because breast
cancer is a diverse group of related problems, I don't expect that
a single "magic bullet" will cure it. However, if there is one area
in which a major earth-shattering change could be made in the
next ten to twenty years, it's in the area of gene manipulation.
In other words, as we continue to locate more and more genes
responsible for breast cancer, we will hopefully see close on the
heels of this research a new arsenal of treatments that directly
target and correct these genetic defects. And while there will
not likely be one single such therapy to eradicate breast cancer,
a group of related gene therapies gleaned from the same tech-
nological advances will likely make a major impact on the
management of this disease. In the meantime, though, no one
would advocate sitting back and waiting for such a breakthrough. Since breast cancer is with us in daunting proportion,

BREAST CANCER SURVIVORS

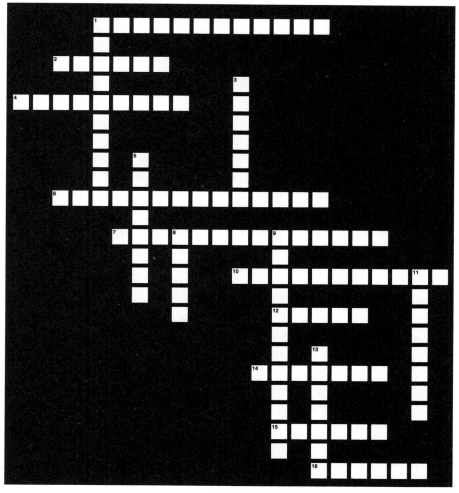

ACROSS

1 Alec, Billy & Stephen's mom
2 *FYI* star _____ Brown
4 First lady
6 *Bosom Buddies*' funny lady
7 She was TV's Julia
10 One of the Angels
12 Newhart's secretary
14 *Bob Newhart Show* costar
15 Pop star from Down Under
16 He followed Nixon

DOWN

1 Pop singer of "You're So Vain" fame
3 The Angels' unseen boss
5 Let's Get _____
8 *Bosom Buddies* star
9 1972 hit by 1 down
11 Where 13 down struck gold
13 Skating star Peggy

it's absolutely vital that we keep developing a wide variety of effective, novel treatments for breast cancer.

◆ MY GRANDMOTHER HAD BREAST CANCER, MY MOTHER HAS IT, AND WHO KNOWS IF I WILL GET IT. I'M SICK AND TIRED OF HEARING THAT SOMEDAY BREAST CANCER WILL BE WIPED OUT. WILL THIS EVER HAPPEN?

While newspaper headlines—and our own hearts and minds—tend to hope for miracle cures, science doesn't often work that way. On the contrary, research is slow and incremental. But before you feel such despair, there are countless examples of breakthroughs in other diseases that you can use as a model for the future course of breast cancer. Consider, for instance, the case of bleeding duodenal ulcers. Today, we think of ulcers as a nuisance—as something that causes discomfort and annoyance, but certainly not as a threat to survival. Well not too many years ago, bleeding ulcers had a mortality rate of 50 percent—that's right, half of people with this condition died, despite emergency surgery and other valiant lifesaving measures. Then, lo and behold, along came a group of drugs called H-2 blockers. These drugs blocked the acid that promotes ulcers, and countless lives were saved. These days it's extremely rare that a doctor would be called upon to operate on a bleeding ulcer. Then, in the mid-1980s, another discovery showed that bacteria are responsible for causing many bleeding ulcers—now antibiotics are curing another large group of patients—so even the H-2 blockers and other acid-fighting medications may become things of the past.

My message is this:

The diagnosis of breast cancer was once considered a death sentence. Then, with the advent of increasingly effective surgical, drug, radiological, and other therapies, and early diagnostic tools, thousands of women began to be saved. We moved from five-, to ten-, to fifteen-year and longer survival rates—and now many women are living well into old age with breast

Just the mention of a cure makes me want to sing:

Rosie with Billy Baldwin
(whose mother is a breast cancer survivor),
to the tune of "Monster Mash"

ROSIE: Ladies, here's a thought this Halloween
If you want to avoid a scary scene
BILLY: It's not quite a treat, but it's not a trick
Grab your breasts and hop on your broomstick . . .
BOTH: Go do the moosh
Go do the booby moosh
The booby moosh
It's just a real quick smoosh
Go do the moosh
Get up off your tush
To do the moosh
Go do the booby moosh!
ROSIE: So take it from your friend Snow White
Have the doc check your left, and then your right!
BILLY: Don't sit there stewing by your cauldron
Get your boobs examined, love Billy Baldwin
BOTH: Go do the moosh
Go do the booby moosh
The booby moosh
This is our friendly push
Go do the moosh
We just refuse to shoosh
Until you moosh
Go do the booby moosh
Wa ooh yeah!

**Rosie with Dr. Deborah Axelrod,
to the tune of "Twinkle Twinkle Little Star"**

ROSIE: Ladies, ladies, here's my wish—
BOTH: That you'll get your boobies squished—
DR. AXELROD: I'm a certified M.D.—
Who wants your jugs to be health-y—
BOTH: Do a monthly self-exam—
'N' for God's sake get a mammogram!—

cancer in their distant past. The many exciting new therapies I will discuss in this chapter may only enhance the already important strides we have made in battling breast cancer—and who knows which one, or ones, will eclipse the others. So instead of looking for a miracle, remember that in medicine, miracles often happen piecemeal. But we are living in a period of unprecedented research activity and promise.

◆ WHAT ARE THESE SO-CALLED MONOCLONAL ANTIBODIES I KEEP READING ABOUT?

Monoclonal antibodies sound very foreign and exotic, but in fact, when you understand how they work, they make a great deal of basic sense. They're also a good example of a "futuristic" form of treatment that is already, to a certain extent, with us today. One

> I think she blew the president . . . and what the hell are you reading?

making the most news these days is a drug called Herceptin. Here's how monoclonal antibodies work:

Every cell in our bodies has receptors on it—receptors for different proteins, or different compounds that the body either produces or is exposed to. Think of the receptors as locks: When the right key is put into that lock, something in the cell is triggered—in the case of cancer, something bad is triggered. The goal of monoclonal antibody therapy is to come up with a fake key—one that very closely resembles the correct key—and to insert that key into the lock on the cell, thereby tricking the cell into thinking that its "needs" have been met, when really the receptor has just been turned off. For example, it has been found that about 25–30 percent of women with breast cancer overexpress a gene for the epidermal growth factor (EGF) receptor, also called HER-2/neu or C-erb B-2, which may be associated with a greater risk of dying from aggressive disease. With monoclonal antibody therapy, a "key" is created that slips into the EGF receptor, effectively turning it off. The result: short-term stabilization of the disease.

So far Herceptin has only been used on women with extensive, metastatic breast cancer—that is, breast cancer that has spread to other sites in the body. The next step, and one that will be critical to the future treatment of breast cancer, is to try this drug in women with early-stage disease, to see if and for how long it can stave off any recurrence or worsening of the disease. It will likely be a few years before Herceptin is given to women with early-stage disease, however, because we need to have more definitive proof of its safety and effectiveness first.

◆ ARE THERE RISKS TO THESE MONOCLONAL ANTIBODIES?

As usual there is no free lunch. Herceptin carries a risk of cardiotoxicity—that is, it can be toxic to the heart—especially when combined with other chemotherapeutic drugs such as Adriamycin (which has its own inherent problems with heart toxicity). There is also the risk of fever, chills, and headache during Herceptin therapy, but generally these side effects are less severe than those caused by other chemotherapy drugs.

The latest studies are looking at Herceptin in combination with a variety of other chemotherapy drugs: taxol, taxanes, cisplatin, and others. These combinations seem to be much safer than the Herceptin-Adriamycin pairing.

◆ WHAT ARE CANCER VACCINES?

There is more than just one "cancer vaccine"—in fact, the word "vaccine" is used rather loosely in the fight against breast cancer, and can refer to several different treatment approaches. For instance, there are vaccines that attempt to work by targeting an error or mutation within a breast cancer cell. And there are vaccines that try to boost the overall immune system, leading the body to attack its own cancer cells. At this point, these approaches are much more effective in laboratory animals than in humans. For example, we can make cancer in mice disappear—but we can't do it in humans yet. It will likely be many more years before any breast cancer vaccine is widely used for the public.

◆ WHAT IS "IMMUNE THERAPY" AND HOW DOES IT FIGHT BREAST CANCER?

Immune treatments for breast cancer involve boosting the body's own natural defenses against cancer cells—so, as I mentioned earlier, one type of cancer vaccine falls into this category. Early on in the course of breast cancer, the body puts up a good fight against the foreign cancer cells. With time, however, the body's immune system often loses the battle, as cancer cells proliferate and spread to other sites. Scientists have found that there are various ways to boost the immune system so that it puts up a stronger, longer fight against cancer— using treatments such as interleukin-2 (IL-2) and interferon. Interleukin-2 is a so-called lymphokine, which means that it triggers the body's own killer cells. Interferon, on the other hand, both kills cancer cells *and* activates the body's own disease-fighting white cells.

MYSTERY MESSAGE

Solve these breast cancer–related puzzles. The letters you insert in the blanks will then form a mystery message (which is truly no mystery at all).

PE__GY FL__MING

SHIRLEY __EMPLE BL__CK

JULIA __ __ILD

KAT__ JA__ __SON

M__RPHY BROWN

CHEMOTHERA__Y

(Answer: GET A CHECKUP)

In the simplest terms, here's how some of these therapies work:

First, natural disease-fighting cells are removed from the woman's body. Then, in the laboratory, they are stimulated in some way (with IL-2, for example) so that they increase both in strength and number. Finally, these new, supercharged immune cells are put back in the woman's body—hopefully to wage a tougher war on cancer cells. The good news is that test tube results show that the immune cells are indeed stimulated. The bad news is that there are some dangerous side effects in humans. *And the question mark hanging out there is whether any of these treatments will translate into a tangible, clinical response in human beings. This we don't know.* I, for one, eagerly await these important scientific results.

◆ **I'VE HEARD ABOUT TRYING TO FIGHT THE "GROWTH FACTORS" IN CANCER CELLS. WHAT'S THIS ALL ABOUT?**

Cancer cells create substances called "growth factors" to help them thrive. These growth factors appear to aid the cancer cell in a variety of ways, including helping it to develop blood vessels, which in turn lead the cells to proliferate and spread throughout the body (more on this later in this chapter). One important area of research aims to find treatments that fight these growth factors. In this instance, one tiny peek into the future is already with us: One of the mechanisms of action of the hormonal drug tamoxifen appears to be blocking some cancer growth factors.

One of the most appealing aspects of such targeted therapy—that is, treatments that home in on the growth factor in a cancer cell, rather than attacking the cell as a whole—is that a great deal of toxicity may be avoided. Treatments that attack whole cancer cells while they are dividing, for example, have the unfortunate side effect of harming the body's *normal* cells as well. This is why so many unpleasant side effects are associated with many chemotherapy drugs. If, on the other hand, we could develop drugs that strike directly at a single factor within a single type of cancer cell, we could spare healthy surrounding cells. The idea can be likened to the "smart bombs" now being used in modern warfare, in which precise, narrow targets are hit, leaving surrounding buildings unscathed.

◆ **THERE WAS SOME MAJOR NEWS RECENTLY ABOUT RESEARCHERS KILLING CANCEROUS TUMORS BY CUTTING OFF THEIR BLOOD SUPPLY. WHAT HAS HAPPENED TO THIS RESEARCH?**

You're asking about a group of treatments called "anti-angiogenesis" drugs—one of the most fascinating and exciting areas of research in the fight against breast cancer. The story of how these treatments work and their potential for the future is an interesting one, but requires a bit of background.

WOULD YOU LIKE SOME ANAGRAMS WITH YOUR MAMMOGRAM, MA'AM?

Here are some fun ways to rearrange the names of some very special breast cancer survivors.

Gloria Steinem . . .

> GELATIN IS MORE
>
> MEAT RELIGIONS
>
> TEAM RELIGIONS
>
> TAME RELIGIONS
>
> MERIT GASOLINE
>
> LIONS EMIGRATE
>
> REGIONAL ITEMS
>
> EELS MIGRATION
>
> ME OIL ANGRIEST

Carly Simon . . .

> MOAN LYRICS
>
> SLIMY ACORN
>
> IS NORMALCY
>
> ON SLIMY CAR
>
> NO AM LYRICS

Shirley Temple Black . . .

> CELEBRATE SILK LYMPH
>
> TILE CLERK BLASPHEMY
>
> YELL TRICK BLASPHEMY
>
> KILL HEM RESPECTABLY
>
> KEY BIRTHPLACE SMELL

Nancy Reagan . . .

> AN ACE GRANNY
>
> RAN AN AGENCY

Marcia Wallace . . .

> CAR AIL LAW CAME

Betty Ford . . .

> FORTY DEBT
>
> DEBT TO FRY

Olivia Newton-John . . .

NO VOW INHALE JOINT

HI JAW NOVEL NOTION

HOT JEAN WON VIOLIN

JOIN INNOVATE HOWL

Carol Baldwin . . .

DO CRAWL IN LAB

RANCID OWL LAB

LILAC DOWN BRA

BLOW CARDINAL

BLOWN RADICAL

Kate Jackson . . .

JACK SENT OAK

ASK NO JACKET

SNEAK TO JACK

Justice O'Connor . . .

REJOIN COCONUTS

ONE JOINT OCCURS

JOINT CONCOURSE

JOIN UNTO SOCCER

Murphy Brown . . .

PURR HYMN BOW

ROW HYMN BURP

Peggy Fleming . . .

PIG MEN FLY EGG

And just to show
I can give and take
the anagramming,

Rosie O'Donnell . . .

SOLD ONE ONLINE

NEON OR DOLLIES

SELL ONE INDOOR

LOON OIL SELLER

Starting about thirty years ago, the field of angiogenesis research started at Children's Hospital in Boston. The scientists were just beginning to understand what controls new blood vessel growth in the body. Why is this relevant to the treatment of breast cancer? Because all so-called solid tumors—breast cancer included—require a blood supply in order to thrive. Without an adequate blood supply, the tumors cannot grow; they cannot spread; and they cannot kill.

As we learned in the diagnosis chapter of this book, breast cancers start out tiny and harmless, and may stay that way, contained in a breast duct, for example, for many years before they start to grow and spread. This is called "in-situ" disease. Researchers know from watching visible tumors, such as skin cancer and cervical cancer, that many years can pass before these tumors switch from a dormant mode to a growing, aggressive mode. At some point, though, the tumors do often switch into another phase in which they begin to recruit their own blood supply. That's when the real trouble begins.

When blood vessels grow around a tumor, the tumor can expand in size: to give you an idea of how big a shift takes place, an in-situ tumor the size of a pencil point may have half a million cells, while one the size of a marble has about a billion cells. And while screening mammography can detect cancers as small as a pencil point, unfortunately many women don't have a mammogram done until their tumor is the size of a marble— long after angiogenesis, or blood vessel growth, has begun.

So the big question is this: Can we cut off the blood supply to a tumor, literally starve it, and thereby render it harmless? In the 1980s, researchers started finding the answers. First, they identified a number of proteins that stimulate the switch from dormant to active blood vessel formation. Then, further research led to the location of a number of such proteins that were directly related to breast cancer. From that point on came exciting discoveries of so-called anti-angiogenesis drugs, which aim to "turn off" these proteins that promote blood vessel growth.

Quietly, but surely, in the early 1990s the first of these drugs went into early scientific animal studies. As of 1999, there are twenty such drugs under study. In animals, these drugs slow tumor growth—and some even shrink pre-existing tumors. The next exciting step in the research came when scientists looked at *several* of these drugs used in concert. Sure enough, just as it was found many years ago that combined chemotherapy drugs work better than single agents, so combined anti–blood vessel drugs seem to work better, and faster, than single ones. Tumors in mice were found to shrink in just a matter of *weeks*, with little or no toxicity. The future question is: Will the same exciting findings apply to humans?

◆ WHAT ABOUT THE USE OF THESE ANTI–BLOOD VESSEL DRUGS IN HUMANS?

This is the next major question, one that only time can answer. The National Cancer Institute formally announced that the first clinical trials of two of these drugs—Endostatin and Angiostatin—will begin in September of 1999. Considering the fact that these agents were discovered in 1997, this is a remarkably fast track for study in humans. The first phase of these studies will determine if the drugs are indeed safe and relatively nontoxic in humans. Then, they will be studied for their effectiveness on human beings. At this point, while the researchers are enormously excited about the potential these drugs may hold, they are cautious: humans are not mice, for one thing. And because breast cancer works in so many tricky ways, it may not be possible to control the disease with a single treatment modality. Right now, most experts' best guess is that these drugs, if found safe and effective, will join other major breast cancer therapies—chemotherapy, radiotherapy, and so on—to create more potent combined weapons against the disease. Also, if all goes according to plan—and fate—these drugs may someday be used to create long periods of remission or to prevent a recurrence.

◆ ARE THESE ANTI-BLOOD VESSEL DRUGS TOXIC IN THE SAME WAY THAT OTHER CHEMOTHERAPY DRUGS CAN BE?

As a group, these drugs seem to have very few toxic effects, because they do not affect the bone marrow or promote hair loss and other common side effects commonly associated with drugs that fight breast cancer. But we need to see the results of longer-term studies in humans to know for sure that these drugs are safe and well tolerated.

◆ IT SEEMS AS IF WE HEAR BIG NEWS ABOUT A POTENTIAL TREATMENT FOR BREAST CANCER, AND THEN THE NEWS FIZZLES OUT AND WE HEAR NOTHING MORE ABOUT IT. WHY DO SO MANY TREATMENTS FAIL TO LIVE UP TO THEIR PROMISE?

This is a very important question, and has a lot to do with the scientific process. The way the media handle medical stories—emphasizing alleged breakthroughs and making major headlines even out of early animal research—people's hopes are raised and dashed time and time again. The fact is, people fail to understand just how much room there is for failure in the course of scientific research. Of hundreds of drugs and other therapies that are tested, only a tiny handful make it to approval and widespread use. There are countless bumps in the road to drug development. One of the biggest is the basic difference between lab rats and human beings. For the purpose of controlled study, lab rats are all identical twins. If researchers used heterogeneous field mice, let's say, they'd have to study enormous numbers to get good results. Well, humans are more like field mice—and a lot more complicated to boot. We not only differ dramatically from other species, we also differ from one another. So, for example, a drug might be extremely effective in rats, but the human liver turns out to destroy the compound. Or maybe mice thrive on the drug, but most humans are allergic to it. Or maybe the problem is much more mundane—say, a drug holds lots of promise, but it can't be shipped because its activity is wiped out by dry ice. Or maybe an exciting new protein sticks to the intravenous tubing and can't be delivered properly. So many treatments fail for these sorts of practical problems—not because the underlying scientific principles are wrong, but because of forces out of scientists' control. When you understand and think about the infinite number of potential roadblocks to scientific research, it's a wonder so many effective treatments *do* eventually make it to the marketplace!

◆ WHILE WE WAIT FOR THE DISCOVERY OF FUTURISTIC BREAST CANCER TREATMENTS, WHAT'S ON THE HORIZON FOR SCREENING?

While there is some limited excitement about the use of tools like MRI and PET scans to aid in the detection of early breast cancers (see page 123–24), most feel that the future of breast cancer screening lies in the genetic code. We may be about ten years away from creating a detailed map of a person's genetic makeup, including a breakdown of the genes that put her at risk for breast cancer. (It could be far longer before this technology is made available to the average woman, however.) I feel that that future of screening will lie in locating those women at greatest risk of getting breast cancer, and then using various preventive treatments to *ward off* the disease. This will mark a major shift from the present, in which detection means catching existing cancers and then treating them.

◆ DO YOU THINK THAT MAINSTREAM AND COMPLEMENTARY TREATMENTS FOR BREAST CANCER WILL SOMEDAY BE CONSIDERED "PARTNERS" IN CARE?

The unfortunate truth of the matter is that the relationship between conventional medicine and complementary therapies is so weak at this point that it could only improve in the future.

There has traditionally been a tall, solid wall between the two "camps"—with suspicion and mistrust on both sides. That said, there is certainly good reason for the two to merge. While conventional therapies aim to fight the cancer itself, complementary therapies care for the person with cancer. In general, I hope the future of medical care will include not just attention to high-tech therapies and exciting genetic breakthroughs, but also a heightened alert to the humane aspects of disease detection and treatment. Certainly the treatment of breast cancer is one area in which attention to the woman's psyche is just as important as the fight against her tumor. The level of anxiety, self-loathing after surgery, long-term fear, depression, and other emotional sequelae to breast cancer and its treatment require special attention and care. Complementary therapies are (along with traditional psychological counseling), in many cases, well equipped to deal with these psychological issues. For instance, massage therapy; stress reduction techniques such as deep breathing, meditation, and yoga; and empowering therapies such as imagery training can all make a big difference in improving a woman's quality of life through breast cancer treatment and beyond.

The future also holds great promise for a better understanding of the role of herbal preparations and nutrition in the fight against breast cancer. For example, the nagging question about the role of estrogenic foods such as soy in relation to breast cancer may become less cloudy in the next several years. Will soy prove to be protective against breast cancer, offering beneficial estrogenic properties but not dangerous ones? Or will we learn that estrogenic foods and plants carry many of the same dangers as their medicinal counterparts? Time, and studies, will tell. However, because these products cannot be patented, there is relatively little money for funding studies on the subject (compared to the financial clout of drug companies, for example). So this lack of money could slow the research process down quite a bit.

Above all else, I sincerely hope the future holds a significant shift in attitudes among various health care practitioners toward the others' treatment approaches: I hope that tradi-

tional practitioners come to realize that those offering complementary therapies are not a threat, but an ally in the effort to
heal whole human beings. And I hope that those who practice
complementary therapies keep open minds about the enormous, proven curative value of conventional medical treatments for cancer.

Notice, by the way, that I have been talking about *complementary* therapies—and not *alternative* therapies. Unproved
therapies that aim to replace, rather than enhance, conventional medicine are sometimes dangerous and often counter-
productive. They should no more represent the future than the
present care of breast cancer.

◆ WHAT STUDIES ARE UNDER WAY NOW THAT HOLD THE MOST EXCITEMENT FOR THE FUTURE?

Many of the issues I've touched on throughout this chapter involve scientific studies that will yield important results for the
treatment of breast cancer—including immunotherapy, vaccine
treatments, and so on. But two very important prevention studies I haven't mentioned yet are the STAR (Study of Tamoxifen
and Raloxifene) trial and the Women's Health Initiative. The
STAR trial, which is about to begin, will pit the hormonal
agents tamoxifen and raloxifene against one another in postmenopausal high-risk women. (More on these drugs can be
found on pages 168–71.) The STAR trial is being conducted by
the National Surgical Adjuvant Breast and Bowel project (NS-
ABP), and I feel that this extremely important research will
translate into easier and clearer choices for many older women
at higher risk of breast cancer in the coming years.

The Women's Health Initiative, supported by the National
Institutes of Health, is another extremely important and impressive series of studies that is trying to assess the effects of
long-term estrogen exposure on the risk of breast disease and
breast cancer, and also the impact of a low-fat diet on breast
cancer risk.

And of course there are countless other vital research proj-

TOP TEN BREAST MOVIES OF ALL TIME

Disney's *A Jug's Life*

A Bra Is Born

Beauty and the Breast

Hello, Dolly (Parton)

Big II

Titty Titty Bang Bang

The sci-fi thriller *Bras Attacks*

Honey, I Blew Up the Tits

Bra Trek V: The Final Brassiere

How the Breast Was Won

Bonus: *TITantic*

ects that I could never begin to list in a single chapter, let alone an entire tome. But rest assured that there is a tremendous body of research under way, focusing on just about every imaginable front in the war against breast cancer.

◆ WHERE DOES FUNDING FOR CANCER RESEARCH COME FROM, AND DOES IT MAKE A BIG DIFFERENCE?

Funding for breast cancer comes from a wide variety of sources, both public and private. The major umbrella organization responsible for a

It comes from your wallet; you can help by opening it.

dramatic shift in public perceptions, actions, and funding on behalf of breast cancer is the National Breast Cancer Coalition (NBCC). Founded as a grassroots organization in 1991, the NBCC now encompasses more than five hundred organizations and represents millions of survivors and their families, women with no history of the disease, as well as professionals from all areas of breast cancer care. Its mission: to eradicate breast cancer through three main approaches: governmental change, scientific research, and consumer advocacy. In the eight short years since its inception, the NBCC has raised federal funding for breast cancer research more than 600 percent, from less than $90 million to more than $600 million. It has led to the creation of a multimillion-dollar breast cancer research project within the Department of Defense. And it has launched a dizzying array of programs, including advocacy training, educational programs, major scientific studies, powerful governmental lobbying campaigns with literally millions of women's support, traveling photographic exhibits, and worldwide breast cancer conferences, among dozens of other major initiatives. So you ask, does the money make a difference? You bet it does. It brings to fruition the great labor and imagination of activists and advocates who dedicate their lives to the long and costly fight against breast cancer. The dollars turn ideas—scientific, legal, and governmental—into reality. And every dollar counts.

Major breast cancer funding from private sources originates with the Komen Foundation, founded by Nancy Brinker in honor of her sister Susan, who died of breast cancer at the age of thirty-six. And another major inspiration in the global fight against breast cancer is Amy Langer, executive director of the National Alliance for Breast Cancer Organizations. Formerly a successful investment banker who developed breast cancer in her thirties, Amy has become a powerful force in terms of boosting breast cancer awareness (especially among the terribly overlooked group of minority women), and has aggressively promoted active education about breast cancer.

◆ I HAVE FRIENDS WHO GATHER A GREAT DEAL OF
BREAST CANCER INFORMATION FROM THE INTERNET.
IS THIS A GOOD SOURCE OF INFORMATION?

That depends. The fact is, the Internet is a vast library of information, and like any other library, it contains a big stew of
terrific—and poor—resources. Because there is no quality control, you can dive into the Web and find all sorts of data about
breast cancer.

How can you know if it's accurate or valuable? Stick to the
sites that are attached to well-regarded, major breast cancer research and advocacy organizations. Not only will they have reliable information, but they will offer appropriate hyperlinks to
other reputable sites as well. For starters, take a look at our Resources section at the end of this book, where we list some
helpful and reliable Internet sites that carry information on
every aspect of breast cancer and its management.

◆ HOW CAN I TAKE PART IN THE FUTURE FIGHT
AGAINST BREAST CANCER?

First, understand that *anyone* can take part in the fight against
breast cancer. While traditionally activists and advocates have
been breast cancer survivors, there is more than enough room
for others in this fight. For instance: family members, friends,
health professionals, or just women who care about protecting
themselves and their daughters from this disease can play a
meaningful role in the war against breast cancer. There are
many different ways to become involved, depending on the
kind of commitment you want to make to the "cause." For instance, even just becoming educated about breast cancer and
telling other women what you have learned makes you part of
the team that fights this disease. You can participate in advocacy training programs, and learn specific ways to lobby governmental officials, for example, to bring about new and better
laws that relate to breast cancer. If you are a survivor, you can
join organizations that will match you to others in similar cir-

cumstances who need your knowledge and support at a difficult point in their diagnostic or treatment process. Or perhaps you would like to become a facilitator in a breast cancer support group. You can help raise money for any number of breast cancer–related projects, from local screening tests in your neighborhood to major national scientific research programs. You can join marches, hikes, bike rides, and protests supporting better funding and increased attention to breast cancer research. You can press your local politicians to support laws that will end discrimination against women with breast cancer in the workplace. And you can fight for laws that will help increase funding for breast cancer screening and other needed resources for lower-income or uninsured women. You can speak to young adult women in schools or in workplace seminars about the risk of breast cancer and the importance of screening. You can donate money to not-for-profit organizations that focus on breast cancer—perhaps a group that helped you, or a loved one, in some way. The list of options is endless—and it is enormously empowering to join hands with the millions of other women and men who share your goal of wiping out this disease.

Ladies, don't forget the men in your life; one of my favorite times in the year is October, Breast Cancer Awareness Month, when I decorate the trees on our block with pink ribbons, and my husband and sons join me in a four-mile walk in Central Park to raise money for breast cancer. The event culminates in a celebration of life, with dancing and enormous energy, and later a candlelight walk in our town. You can create a life-affirming celebration of this kind in your city or town, too. Know this: You are needed. Just announce that you are ready to help, and you're on your way.

BREAST CANCER—THE FUTURE

```
I  B  S  Z  T  I  D  K  J  D  G  I  S  P  I  A  J  T  W  E
Z  N  N  S  J  G  T  J  Z  Q  S  I  O  Z  F  I  V  W  S  I
R  K  D  S  E  M  G  R  D  I  A  W  V  N  H  H  N  B  E  M
K  M  H  Q  X  S  H  D  D  S  G  Y  W  C  A  A  O  R  N  S
D  Z  G  E  N  E  S  V  U  P  C  G  M  H  V  N  D  T  I  Z
F  K  I  I  S  Z  K  X  X  D  N  R  W  E  L  E  V  G  C  U
O  I  Q  B  F  F  E  X  M  A  M  N  H  M  R  U  M  I  C  G
X  R  X  P  H  S  J  Z  Y  P  X  E  E  O  L  T  P  M  A  G
L  C  G  C  P  M  K  J  I  E  H  D  E  P  A  K  O  X  V  N
V  P  B  V  C  V  I  N  S  A  U  J  D  R  P  F  V  G  B  V
N  K  V  E  C  K  V  K  X  R  L  N  E  E  B  Y  E  J  Y  H
F  H  W  M  C  B  J  U  F  M  X  P  G  V  S  U  W  M  P  P
P  Y  F  T  U  V  S  C  M  G  W  P  B  E  B  O  B  K  Y  H
J  V  A  P  N  M  L  A  R  Z  Y  K  O  N  H  R  R  N  A  Q
X  P  P  E  W  Q  V  K  M  L  K  E  G  T  B  N  Z  V  K  H
M  O  N  O  C  L  O  N  A  L  A  N  T  I  B  O  D  I  E  S
V  N  Q  G  K  M  T  N  B  M  Q  J  S  O  J  K  X  S  I  U
C  U  N  Z  V  L  M  D  N  R  M  N  N  G  A  Y  I  B  R
B  N  S  W  A  A  B  M  A  D  J  K  N  K  Y  N  X  H  X  L
J  T  V  X  W  B  G  B  V  Q  C  G  P  V  E  C  S  Y  U  I
```

Find and circle the following words:

CHEMOPREVENTION   MONOCLONAL ANTIBODIES
GENES   VACCINES

AFTERWORD

Okay, you've done it. Soup to nuts. What exactly did you do? Well, for starters you bought the book—all the profits go to charity. Not bad. Then maybe you got a few questions answered, thought of some new questions to ask—even laughed a little. I know you picked up a few new boob names.

You learned some pretty interesting facts: What a lump feels like, what to eat, the importance of family history (just to name a few), the things we need to know to get us well, and keep us well. Bottom line, I hope we conveyed the power of sharing information and educating ourselves.

There are few things in life as terrifying and isolating as a breast cancer diagnosis. But the truth is, you are not alone, and you are not without resources. There are legions of us who are your Bosom Buddies. Armed with knowledge, we have power and we have hope.

So now you've read the whole book—what do you do? Put it on your shelf and hope you never need it. Buy a copy for your sister, mother, friend, neighbor—whoever you think should read it. Make a new Bosom Buddy. When information is the gold standard, it's easy to make everybody rich.

RESOURCES

The majority of the following listings have been excerpted from the NABCO *Breast Cancer Resource List*, ©1999, Annual Edition, with permission from the National Alliance of Breast Cancer Organizations (NABCO), New York, NY, (888) 80-NABCO, www.nabco.org. To obtain a copy of the NABCO *Breast Cancer Resource List*, and for more information about breast cancer, contact NABCO.

GENERAL INFORMATION ABOUT BREAST CANCER

ASK NABCO^{SM} is NABCO's online column, which answers common questions about risk, detection, and treatment of breast cancer. On NABCO's Web site at www.nabco.org, or call (888) 80-NABCO to order a hard copy version of one or more features. To submit questions, e-mail asknabco@aol.com.

BREAST CANCER FACTS & FIGURES 1997/1998 (8610.98). A booklet containing the most up-to-date statistics on breast cancer, including incidence, survival, and trends. ACS (800) ACS-2345 or www.cancer.org.

BREAST CANCER: THE COMPLETE GUIDE by Yashar Hirshaut, M.D. and Peter Pressman, M.D. (Bantam, New York, 1996 edition, paperback $14.95). An easy-to-follow resource providing up-to-date medical information and practical advice on breast cancer, from suspicion of disease through diagnosis, treatment, and follow-up care. Dr. Pressman is a member of NABCO's Medical Advisory Board; the foreword is by Amy Langer, executive director of NABCO. 334 pages. Bookstores. (*Note:* A new edition is expected in late 1999.)

DR. SUSAN LOVE'S BREAST BOOK by Susan M. Love, M.D. with Karen Lindsey (Addison Wesley, Reading, MA, 1995 revised edition, paperback $17.00). A breast surgeon discusses all conditions of the breast, from benign to malignant. The author's viewpoint on treatment options and controversies is clearly presented in a friendly, accessible style. A good general reference. 657 pages. Bookstores.

UNDERSTANDING BREAST CANCER TREATMENT (July 1998). This booklet contains lists of questions that will help a patient talk to her doctor about breast cancer. Breast cancer topics covered include: early detection, diagnosis, treatment, adjuvant therapy, and reconstruction. 72 pages. NCI's Cancer Information Service (800) 4-CANCER or rex.nci.nih.gov.

CANCER FACTS & FIGURES—1999 (5508.99 LE, January 1999). An annual publication of the American Cancer Society, this booklet gives the latest incidence and mortality statistics and trends by site and geographical location. 32 pages. ACS, (800) ACS-2345 or www.cancer.org.

WHAT YOU NEED TO KNOW ABOUT CANCER (1998). The NCI's overview booklet about cancer—what it is, who is at risk, and common treatments. 34 pages. NCI's CIS, (800) 4-CANCER.

BREAST CANCER TREATMENT GUIDELINES FOR PATIENTS, Version 1, January 1999 (99-50M-No.9405-HCP) American Cancer Society and National Comprehensive Cancer Network (800) ACS-2345, (888) 909-NCCN.

PERSONAL STORIES

BREAST CANCER? LET ME CHECK MY SCHEDULE! edited by Peggy McCarthy and Jo An Loren (Westview Press, Boulder, CO, 1997, paperback, $14.00). Ten professional women (including NABCO's Amy Langer) share their wisdom and experience about what it means to live with breast cancer. 235 pages. Order from Westview Press, (800) 386-5656.

THE CANCER JOURNALS by Audre Lorde (Aunt Lute Books, San Francisco, 1980, paperback, $7.00). Reflections on her breast cancer by the late black lesbian poet. 77 pages. Available from Aunt Lute Books, PO Box 410687, San Francisco, CA 94141, (415) 826-1300.

THE CLIMB OF MY LIFE by Laura Evans (Harper, San Francisco, 1996, $22.00). The author traces her experience from the time she was diagnosed with breast cancer in 1990 to 1995, when she led sixteen other breast cancer survivors in a climb to the summit of the highest mountain in the Western Hemisphere. Laura Evans is the founder of Expedition Inspiration. Bookstores.

FIRST, YOU CRY by Betty Rollin (Harper Paperbacks, New York, 1993 edition, paperback, $5.50). The newest edition of the first "mass-market" personal account, the pathbreaking autobiographical account of her experience with breast cancer in the 1970s by the NBC correspondent and NABCO Honorary Board member. 213 pages. Bookstores.

NOT NOW . . . I'M HAVING A NO HAIR DAY: HUMOR AND HEALING FOR PEOPLE WITH CANCER by Christine Clifford, illustrated by Jack Lindstrom (Pfeifer-Hamilton, Duluth, MN, 1996, $9.95 plus $4.45 shipping). Using her own experience with breast cancer, the author shows how the power of laughter and positive thinking promote recovery and growth. 144 pages. Order from The Cancer Club, 6533 Limerick Drive, Edina, MN 55439, (800) 586-9062, www.cancerclub.com.

PORTRAITS OF HOPE by Nora Feller and Marcia Stevens Sherrill (Smithmark Publishers, New York, NY, 1998, $24.95). Fifty-two inspirational survivors are profiled by Ms. Sherrill and their color portraits are photographed by Ms. Feller. The two-volume set includes a journal for thoughts and notes. Includes a foreword by Rosie O'Donnell, and information about breast cancer from NABCO. 112 pages plus journal. Bookstores.

THE RACE IS RUN ONE STEP AT A TIME: MY PERSONAL STRUGGLE AND EVERY WOMAN'S GUIDE TO TAKING CHARGE OF BREAST CANCER by Nancy Brinker with Catherine McEvily Harris (Summit Publishing Group, Texas, 1995, paperback, $13.95 plus shipping). Ms. Brinker, founder of the Susan G. Komen Foundation and Race for the Cure®, and a NABCO cofounder, discusses the latest advances in detection, treatment options, and statistics, along with her own powerful story. All royalties from the book are donated to the Komen Foundation. 270 pages. Bookstores or the Komen Foundation, (800) I'M AWARE. (Audiotape version available).

HOW TO FIND A QUALIFIED MAMMOGRAPHY PROVIDER

• For the nearest FDA-certified mammography provider, or to check the status of your imaging center, call the NCI's CIS at (800) 4-CANCER.

THINGS TO KNOW ABOUT QUALITY MAMMOGRAMS (AHCPR Publication No. 95-0634). Still current, this consumer pamphlet details the U.S. government's Agency for Health Care Policy and Research recommendations for getting the best mammogram. Also available in Spanish. Up to 200 copies free of charge. Agency for Health Care Policy and Research, Publications Clearinghouse, PO Box 8547, Silver Spring, MD 20907, (800) 358-9295.

GENETICS, RISK FACTORS, AND BENIGN BREAST DISEASE

CANCER FACTS QUESTIONS AND ANSWERS: THE BREAST CANCER PREVENTION TRIAL (1998). This fact sheet answers common questions about The Breast Cancer Prevention Trial including its design, results, and significance for women. 9 pages. Available at no charge from the National Cancer Institute, (800) 4-CANCER.

THE NATIONAL CANCER INSTITUTE'S BREAST CANCER RISK ASSESSMENT TOOL. The "Risk Disk" (September 1998) is free from the NCI and serves as an interactive patient education tool to help assess an individual's risk of developing breast cancer. NCI, (800) 4-CANCER.

QUESTIONS AND ANSWERS ABOUT BREAST CALCIFICATIONS (95-3198, 1995). This brief brochure discusses calcifications of the breast, their significance, and what can be done about them. 3 pages. NCI's CIS, (800) 4-CANCER.

UNDERSTANDING GENE TESTING (96-3905, NIH publication No. 97-3905, January 1997, 31 pages). This easy-to-understand guide provides readers with basic information and addresses issues raised when considering testing under managed care. 30 pages. Order from NIC's CIS, (800) 4-CANCER.

• The Family Cancer Risk Counseling and Genetic Testing Directory offers a listing of cancer risk counseling resources and genetic testing providers across the country. This online service is found on CancerNet™, the Web site of the National Cancer Institute (NCI), and can be assessed by visiting the Web site at cancernet.nci.nih.gov/wwwprot/genetic/genesrch.shtml (no "www" is needed). The directory is searchable by name, city, state, country, and type of cancer or cancer gene.

TREATMENT

CANCERFAX®. This service allows access to NCI's Physician's Data Query (PDQ) system (see entry below) via fax machine, 24 hours a day, 7 days a week, at no charge other than the charge for the fax call. Two versions of the treatment information are available: one for health care professionals and the other for patients, family, or the general public. Information also available in Spanish. To obtain instructions and list of necessary codes, call (301) 402-5874. If there are problems with the fax, call (800) 624-7890, or obtain code information by phone through the Cancer Information Service at (800) 4-CANCER or on the Web, cancernet.nci.nih.gov.

CANCER TRIALS is a new, updated NCI resource on the Web that is all about clinical trials for cancer. It is easy to use and navigate, and was designed to help users find and choose a treatment trial, and offers news about research discoveries. Go to cancertrials.nic.nih.gov (no "www" is necessary).

COMMUNITY CLINICAL ONCOLOGY PROGRAM (CCOP). These 75 medical centers in 30 states have been selected by the National Cancer Institute to participate in a program to introduce the newest clinical protocols and to accrue patients to clinical trials. NCI's CIS, (800) 4-CANCER or www.nci.nih.gov.

PDQ (PHYSICIAN DATA QUERY). The computerized cancer database of the NCI, providing information on treatment, organizations, doctors involved in cancer care, and a listing of more than 1,500 clinical trials that are open to patient accrual. Access by computer equipped with a modem and by fax. For more information, call the NCI's CIS at (800) 4-CANCER or on the Internet, cancernet.nci.nih.gov (no "www" is necessary).

TAKING PART IN CLINICAL TRIALS: WHAT CANCER PATIENTS NEED TO KNOW (98-4250, 1998). A booklet designed for patients who are considering participating in cancer treatment trials. It explains clinical trials to patients in easy-to-understand terms and gives information that will help them to reach an appropriate decision. Includes a glossary. 18 pages. Also available in Spanish. NCI's CIS, (800) 4-CANCER.

• The NCI's PDQ database offers extensive information on treatment trials. Information is available by phone at (800) 4-CANCER, fax at (301) 402-5874, or on the Web at cancertrials.nci.nih.gov. You may request English or Spanish, and formats designed for patients and for professionals.

◆ ◆

FINDING A DOCTOR

• Ask your family doctor or gynecologist for a referral, or ask NABCO. Your doctor can also contact the American Society of Clinical Oncology at (703) 299-0150 or www.asco.org to be referred to local surgical oncologists who are ASCO members. The American Board of Medical Specialties at (800) 776-2378 can verify a physician's board certification by specialty and year, and will refer callers to local board-certified doctors. Many state health departments now maintain a "Consumer Information" section of their Web sites that includes an updated, alphabetical listing of state physicians who have been cited for professional misconduct.

• Call the National Cancer Institute's Cancer Information Service at (800) 4-CANCER for the names of NCI-affiliated treatment centers in your state, including members of the NCI's CCOP program. If none of these centers is conveniently located, call the Department of Surgery at the nearest one and ask for a local referral.

• For referrals to a plastic surgeon for corrective or reconstructive procedures, call the American Society of Plastic and Reconstructive Surgeons' referral service at (800) 635-0635 and a list of several local board-certified plastic surgeons will be mailed to you.

COMPLEMENTARY ALTERNATIVE TREATMENTS

NATIONAL CENTER FOR COMPLEMENTARY AND ALTERNATIVE MEDICINE at the National Institutes of Health investigates alternative medical treatments, helps integrate effective treatment into mainstream medical practice, and offers information packages. NCCAM Clearinghouse, PO Box 8218, Silver Spring, MD, 20907-8218, (888) 644-6226, fax (301) 495-4957, nccam.nih.gov.

THE AMERICAN CANCER SOCIETY has statements providing details on each of the treatment methods included in ACS's brochure *Questionable Methods of Cancer Management* (1993, 3023). Available at local division offices, call (800) ACS-2345 or at www.cancer.org.

THE ALTERNATIVE MEDICINE HOMEPAGE is a Web site that links to information sources about alternative and complementary therapies at www.pitt.edu/~cbw/altm.html.

CHEMOTHERAPY

CHEMOTHERAPY AND YOU: A GUIDE TO SELF-HELP DURING TREATMENT (97-1136, 1997). A booklet, in question-and-answer format, addressing concerns of patients receiving chemotherapy. Emphasis is on explanation, self-help, and participation during treatment. Includes a glossary of terms. 56 pages. NCI's CIS, (800) 4-CANCER.

HELPING YOURSELF DURING CHEMOTHERAPY: 4 STEPS FOR PATIENTS (94-3701, 1994). This easy-to-read brochure suggests four steps to follow during chemotherapy treatment. 12 pages. NCI's CIS, (800) 4-CANCER.

UNDERSTANDING CHEMOTHERAPY (1998, 4458). This booklet provides a brief introduction to chemotherapy, its benefits and side effects. ACS, (800) ACS-2345.

PHARMACEUTICAL COMPANY
BREAST CANCER PATIENT ASSISTANCE PROGRAMS

The following listing of selected reimbursement assistance programs for oncology-related products was excerpted with permission from *Oncology Issues*, a publication of the Association of Community Cancer Centers (July–August 1998).

Amgen Inc.
Amgen Reimbursement Hotline
Monday–Friday, 9 am–5 pm, EST
(800) 272-9376
* For EPOGEN (epoetin alfa), NEUPOGEN (filgrastim).

Bristol-Myers Squibb Oncology/Immunology
Reimbursement Assistance Program (RAP)
Monday–Friday, 8:30 am–5 pm, EST
(800) 872-8718
* For BCNU (carmustine), CISPLATIN (plastinol), CYTOXAN (cyclophosphamide), MEGACE (megestrol), TAXOL (paclitaxel).

Genentech, Inc.
Single Point of Contact (SPOC)
9 am–8 pm, EST
(888) 249-4918; Fax (888) 249-4919
* For HERCEPTIN (trastuzumab).

Glaxo Wellcome Inc.
Oncology Reimbursement Hotline
Monday–Friday, 9 am–5 pm, EST
(800) 745-2967
also, Drug Information Services
(800) 334-0089
* For WELLCOVORIN (leucovorin), NAVELBINE (vinorelbine tartrate).

IMMUNEX Corporation
Immunex Reimbursement Hotline
Monday–Friday, 8:30 am–5:30 pm, EST
(800) 321-4669;
Fax (800) 944-3184 (24 hrs.)
* For LEUCOVORIN CALCIUM (leucovorin), LEUKINE (sargramostim), METHOTREXATE, NOVANTRONE (mitoxantrone).

Lilly Oncology
Lilly Cares
Monday–Friday, 8 am–5 pm, EST
(800) 545-6962
* For VELBAN (vinblastine), ONCOVIN (vincristine).

Merck & Co., Inc.
The Merck Patient Assistance Program
Monday–Friday, 8 am–12 am, EST
(800) 994-2111
* For DECADRON (dexamethasone).

Novartis Pharmaceuticals Corp.
AREDIA (pamidronate disodium)
Reimbursement Hotline
Monday–Friday, 9 am–5 pm, EST
(800) 282-7630

FEMARA (letrozole) Reimbursement Hotline
Monday–Friday, 9 am–5 pm, EST
(888) 508-8087

Ortho Biotech Inc.
Comprehensive Reimbursement, Customer Service, and Clinical Support
Monday–Friday, 9 am–8 pm, EST
(800) 553-3851
* For PROCRIT (epoetin alpha).

Pharmacia & Upjohn Company
Pharmacia & Upjohn Oncology Reimbursement Assistance Program
Monday–Friday, 9 am–5 pm, EST
(800) 808-9111; Fax (703) 706-5925
* For ADRIAMYCIN (doxorubicin), PROVERA/DEPO-PROVERA (medroxyprogesterone), ZINECARD (dexrazoxane).

Rhône-Poulenc Rorer Oncology's
PACT HOTLINE
Providing Access to Chemotherapy
Monday–Friday, 8:30 am–6 pm, EST
(800) 996-6626; Fax (800) 996-6627
* For TAXOTERE (docetaxel).

Roche Laboratories Inc.
Oncoline
Monday–Friday, 9 am–5 pm, EST
(800) 443-6676
* For XELODA (capecitabine), 5-FU (fluorouracil).

Roxane Laboratories, Inc.
Patient Assistance Program
Monday–Friday, 8 am–6 pm, EST
(800) 274-8651
* For ROXANOL (morphine), ROXICODONE (oxycodone).

Schering Sales Corporation
Schering's Commitment to Care
Monday–Friday, 9 am–5 pm, EST
(800) 521-7157
* For FARESTON (toremifine).

Sequus Pharmaceutical, Inc.
SEQUUS Reimbursement Programs
Monday–Friday, 9 am–5 pm, CST
(800) 375-1658
* For DOXIL (doxorubicin).

SmithKline Beecham Oncology
Reimbursement HELPline
Monday–Friday, 6 am–5 pm, PST
(800) 699-3806
* For KYTRIL (granisetron hydrochloride).

Zeneca Pharmaceuticals
Patient Assistance Program
Monday–Friday, 9 am–4 pm, EST
(800) 424-3727
* For NOLVADEX (tamoxifen citrate).

ZOLADEX (goserelin)
Reimbursement Hotline
Monday–Friday, 8:30 am–4:30 pm, EST
(800) 400-4140, Option 1, Option 3

* *

BREAST RECONSTRUCTION

BREAST IMPLANTS: AN INFORMATION UPDATE (U.S. Food and Drug Administration). Contains information about silicone gel–filled and saline-filled breast implants for reconstruction and augmentation. Covers issues such as FDA regulation, scientific studies, alternatives to breast implants, and answers to frequently asked questions. For more information, call (800) 532-4440 or www.fda.gov/oca/breastimplants/bitac.html.

BREAST RECONSTRUCTION AFTER MASTECTOMY (1996, 4630). Describes types of surgery with photographs and drawings, and gives answers to commonly asked questions as well as a glossary of terms. 20 pages. ACS, (800) ACS-2345.

RECURRENCE AND METASTATIC BREAST CANCER

ADVANCED BREAST CANCER: A GUIDE TO LIVING WITH METASTATIC DISEASE by Musa Mayer (O'Reilley & Associates, Inc., Sebastopol, CA, 1998, $19.95). This updated, retitled edition of the author's 1997 *Holding Tight, Letting Go,* helps women lead everyday lives while coping with advanced disease. Includes information on treatment options, managing side effects and pain, finding support, and handling emotional issues, along with personal stories of men and women living with metastatic breast cancer. Contains a good resource section. Bookstores.

HOSPICE RESOURCES. Organizations to consult for information about hospice care and referrals to local hospice programs include Hospice Foundation of America, 20001 S Street, NW, Suite 300, Washington, DC 20009, (202) 638-5419 or www.hospicefoundation.org; Hospice Link, 190 Westbrook Rd., Essex, CT 06426-0713, (800) 331-1620; or in Alaska and Connecticut, (203) 767-1620; and National Hospice Organization, 1901 North Moore St, Suite 901, Arlington, VA 22209, (800) 658-8898 or www.nho.org.

MANAGING CANCER PAIN (1994). Still current, this consumer booklet details the U.S. government's Agency for Health Care Policy and Research's guidelines for treating cancer pain. Available at no charge from AHCPR Publications Clearinghouse, PO Box 8547, Silver Spring, MD 20907-8547, (800) 358-9295. Call (301) 594-1364 for more information.

QUESTIONS AND ANSWERS ABOUT PAIN CONTROL: A GUIDE FOR PEOPLE WITH CANCER AND THEIR FAMILIES (95-3264, 1993). Discusses pain control using both medical and nonmedical methods. The emphasis is on explanation, self-help, and patient participation. 76 pages. ACS, (800) ACS-2345 or NCI's CIS, (800) 4-CANCER.

HOW YOU LOOK AND FEEL

LOOK GOOD . . . FEEL BETTER is a public service program sponsored by the Cosmetic, Toiletry and Fragrance Association Foundation in partnership with ACS and the National Cosmetology Association. It helps women recovering from temporary or permanent cancer manage changes in their appearance resulting from cancer treatment. The program's print and videotape materials are available both to patients and to health professionals. Instructional sessions run by ACS are offered in a number of locations. Materials are also available in Spanish. Call (800) 395-LOOK or (800) ACS-2345.

"TLC" is a catalog created by the American Cancer Society for female cancer survivors. It offers products that help women cope with treatment. Medicare reimbursement for the products is available. For a copy of the catalog, call (800) 850-9445.

Y-ME PROSTHESIS AND WIG BANK. Y-ME National Breast Cancer Organization maintains a prosthesis and wig bank for women in financial need. If the appropriate size is available, Y-ME will mail a wig and/or breast prosthesis anywhere in the country. The organization's hotline is staffed with breast cancer survivors and is a 24-hour service. A nominal handling fee is requested. Call (800) 221-2141.

• For a listing of the sixteen boutiques around the country that sell breast cancer–related products, go to www.breastdoc.com.

FINANCIAL, INSURANCE, AND LEGAL ISSUES

CANCER TREATMENTS YOUR INSURANCE SHOULD COVER (April 1995). Brochure that describes standard and investigational treatments that should be covered, and what to do if reimbursement is denied. Eight pages. Order from The Association of Community Cancer Centers, 11600 Nebel Street, Suite 201, Rockville, MD 20852, (301) 984-9496.

THE CONSUMER'S GUIDE TO DISABILITY INSURANCE (1995). A comprehensive guide to understanding disability insurance. 12 pages. Health Insurance Association of America (HIAA), (202) 824-1600.

U.S. DEPARTMENT OF LABOR, PENSION, AND WELFARE BENEFITS ADMINISTRATION describes the Health Insurance Portability and Accountability Act of 1996. This service also publishes *Questions and Answers: Recent Changes in Healthcare Law*, a summary guide to HIPAA. Call (800) 998-7542.

WHAT CANCER SURVIVORS NEED TO KNOW ABOUT HEALTH INSURANCE (1995) provides a clear understanding of health insurance and how to receive maximum reimbursement for claims. 29 pages. Single copies available free. Order from the National Coalition for Cancer Survivorship, (888) 937-6227. The NCCS also publishes *A Cancer Survivor's Almanac*, which contains useful information about insurance coverage.

• You may be eligible for Supplemental Security Income (SSI) and/or Social Security benefits. While receiving SSI, you could also be eligible for food stamps and Medicaid. For information, and to set up a time to speak with a representative who can help you get started, ask your hospital social worker or call the Social Security Administration at (800) 772-1213.

• Medicare beneficiaries should obtain a copy of *Your Medicare Handbook* from the HCFA, the federal agency that administers Medicare. Write to the Health Care Finance Administration, 6325 Security Blvd., Baltimore, MD 21207, or call the National Medicare Hotline at (800) 638-6833, or the Social Security Administration at (800) 772-3736.

• The American Cancer Society office in your area can provide information on local sources of financial assistance. Check your telephone directory for the number.

THE NATIONAL INSURANCE CONSUMER HELPLINE is a hotline that answers consumer questions, and offers problem-solving support and printed materials including information on life and property casualty insurance. Open 8:00 a.m. to 8:00 p.m. Eastern Standard Time, Monday through Friday, (800) 942-4242.

STATE LAWS RELATING TO BREAST CANCER (CDC, March 1998). The Centers for Disease Control and Prevention has published a summary of statutes across the country related to breast cancer. Available from the CDC at (770) 488-4751 or www.cdc.gov.

• Cancer Care, Inc., based in New York City, offers a toll-free counseling line with support services, education, information, referrals, and financial assistance. (800) 813-HOPE.

YOUR LOVED ONES

MALE PARTNERS:

A SIGNIFICANT JOURNEY: BREAST CANCER SURVIVORS AND THE MEN WHO LOVE THEM is a videotape that addresses breast cancer's effect on a couple's communication, intimacy, and sexuality. Available from the American Cancer Society, (800) 850-9445.

WHEN THE WOMAN YOU LOVE HAS BREAST CANCER (1994). A Y-ME booklet that helps partners give emotional support to their loved ones. Single copies available free, bulk orders available on request. Call (800) 221-2141.

LESBIANS:

MAUTNER PROJECT FOR LESBIANS WITH CANCER is a volunteer organization dedicated to helping lesbians with cancer, as well as their partners and caregivers. The pamphlet *Lesbians and Cancer* provides early detection information and addresses issues for lesbians. Available at no cost in English or Spanish from the Mautner Project, 1707 L Street NW, Suite 500, Washington, DC 20036, (202) 332-5536, www.mautnerproject.org.

CHILDREN:

HANDBOOK FOR MOTHERS SUPPORTING DAUGHTERS WITH BREAST CANCER (1995) gives practical advice and sources of information to the mothers of women with breast cancer. 26 pages. Order from Mothers Supporting Daughters with Breast Cancer, 21710 Bayshore Road, Chestertown, MD 21620-4401, (410) 778-1982, www.azstarnet.com/~pud/msdbc.

◆ ◆ ◆ ◆ ◆ ◆ ◆ ◆ ◆ ◆ ◆ ◆ ◆ ◆ ◆ ◆ ◆ ◆ ◆ ◆

AMERICAN CANCER SOCIETY offers two free pamphlets for families with a parent who has cancer. *Helping Children Understand: A Guide for a Parent with Cancer* and *It Helps to Have Friends* are available free of charge from the ACS by calling (800) ACS-2345.

HOW TO HELP CHILDREN THROUGH A PARENT'S SERIOUS ILL-NESS by Kathleen McCue, MA, CCLS with Ron Bonn (St. Martin's Press, NY, 1994, $18.95). This practical guide explains children's special needs when a parent is seriously ill. Provides guidelines, advice, and real-life examples to help parents and other caregivers help children during this stressful time. 221 pages. Bookstores.

KEMOSHARK by H. Elizabeth King and illustrated by Diane Willford Steele (1995). A colorfully illustrated booklet to help children understand chemotherapy when their parents are undergoing treatment. 14 pages. Order from KID-SCOPE, 3400 Peachtree Road, Suite 703, Atlanta, GA 30326, (404) 233-0001, www.kidscope.org.

MIRA'S MONTH by Deborah Weinstein-Stern. When Stern's breast cancer recurred, she wrote this book for her four-year-old daughter, to help her cope while Mom was in the hospital for a month. It chronicles the events and feelings that a child experiences from the day she learns of her mother's cancer, to the day her mother returns home from the hospital. 38 pages. Available for $5.00 from the Blood and Marrow Transplant Newsletter at (847) 831-1913 or fax (847) 831-1943.

MOMS DON'T GET SICK by Pat Brack with Ben Brack (Melius Publishing, Pierre, SD, 1990, $10.95). Told from a breast cancer patient's point of view and that of her ten-year-old son, this story covers more than a year in the life of the Brack home and is "a story of anger, pain, hope, and joy." 106 pages. (800) 882-5171.

MY MOM HAS BREAST CANCER: A GUIDE FOR FAMILIES (1996, 33 minutes). A KIDSCOPE, Inc., video for parents and children about coping with a mother's breast cancer diagnosis. Structured as interviews with six breast cancer survivors and their young children. Order from KIDSCOPE, 3400 Peachtree Road, Suite 703, Atlanta, GA 30326, (404) 233-0001, www.kidscope.org.

THE PAPER CHAIN by Claire Blake, Eliza Blanchard, and Kathy Parkinson (Health Press, 1998). For children ages three to eight, this book relays the emotions of two young boys whose mom has breast cancer. The story includes the mother going to the hospital, having less energy for her sons, and their changed lifestyle. The book encourages hope and warm feelings. 32 pages. Bookstores or call (800) 643-BOOK.

OUR FAMILY HAS CANCER, TOO! by Christine Clifford (Pfeifer-Hamilton Publishers, Duluth, MN, 1997, $6.95 plus $2.45 shipping). For children ages five to 14, this book talks about one child's struggle to understand and cope with his mother's cancer. Illustrated with cartoons. 64 pages. Available from The Cancer Club, 6533 Limerick Drive, Edina, MN 55439, (800) 586-9062, www.cancerclub.com or bookstores.

SAMMY'S MOMMY HAS CANCER by Sherry Kohlenberg (Magination Press, NY, 1993, paperback, $8.95). The author, who was diagnosed with breast cancer when she was 34 and her son was 18 months old, offers parents a thoughtful and sensitive way to explain breast cancer to a child. Ms. Kohlenberg was a co-founder of the Virginia Breast Cancer Foundation and died in 1993. 32 pages. Bookstores or (800) 825-3089. In Pennsylvania (215) 625-8900.

TALKING ABOUT YOUR CANCER: A PARENT'S GUIDE TO HELPING CHILDREN COPE. A videotape from the Fox Chase Cancer Center that helps parents with cancer explain their diagnosis to their children, offering reassurance to families struggling with a new diagnosis and information for those already coping with cancer. 18 minutes. $29.95 plus $5.00 shipping. Call (215) 728-2668.

WHEN A PARENT HAS CANCER: A GUIDE TO CARING FOR YOUR CHILDREN with **BECKY AND THE WORRY CUP** by Wendy S. Harpham, M.D. (HarperCollins Publishers, 1997, $24.00). The author, a lymphoma survivor, presents sensitive and practical advice to help children understand and cope with a parent's diagnosis of cancer. 164 pages. An illustrated children's book is included that tells the poignant story of Becky, a seven-year-old girl and her experiences with her mother's cancer. 46 pages. Bookstores.

WHEN SOMEONE IN YOUR FAMILY HAS CANCER (96-2685, 1995). A booklet written for the young person whose parent has cancer. It describes what cancer is, its treatment, and its emotional impact on family relationships. Includes a glossary of cancer-related terms. 28 pages. NCI's CIS, (800) 4-CANCER.

Cancer Care, Inc. offers the Helping Children Cope Program of support groups and telephone counseling for children whose parent has cancer. For more information, call (800) 813-HOPE, or www.cancercare.org.

American Cancer Society runs a six-session program, Kids Count Too, for children ages three through teens coping with a parent's cancer. Call (800) ACS-2345 to find the program nearest you, or visit www.cancer.org.

Susan G. Komen Foundation runs Kids Konnected, a support group for children whose mothers have breast cancer. To learn more, call (800) 462-9273, or www.kidskonnected.org.

CARINGKIDS is an Internet support group for children who know someone who is ill. It offers a monitored, open forum where kids may exchange information, share their feelings, and make friends with other kids dealing with similar issues. To subscribe, go to oncolink.upenn.edu/forms/listserv.html.

NCI-DESIGNATED CANCER CENTERS

The institutions listed below have been recognized as Cancer Centers by the National Cancer Institute. They receive financial support from the NCI and from many other sources. The list is current as of early 1999.

ALABAMA
University of Alabama at Birmingham
Comprehensive Cancer Center*
Wallace Tumor Institute
Room 237
1824 Sixth Avenue South
Birmingham, AL 35294-3300
(205) 975-8222, (800) 822-0933

ARIZONA
University of Arizona Cancer Center*
1515 North Campbell Avenue
P.O. Box 245024
Tucson, AZ 85724
(520) 626-6044
(800) 622-COPE

*Indicates Comprehensive Cancer Center
**Indicates Clinical Cancer Center

CALIFORNIA

USC/Norris Comprehensive Cancer Center & Hospital*
1441 Eastlake Ave.
Los Angeles, CA 90033-0800
(800) 872-2273
(323) 865-3000

Jonsson Comprehensive Cancer Center*
University of California at Los Angeles
Box 951781
684 Factor Bldg.
Los Angeles, CA 90095-1781
(800) 825-2631
(310) 825-5268

City of Hope National Medical Center*
Beckman Research Institute
1500 East Duarte Road
Duarte, CA 91010-3000
(800) 826-4673
(800) 678-9990/(626) 359-8111

Chao Family Comprehensive Cancer Center*
University of California at Irvine
Building 23, Route 81
101 The City Drive
Orange, CA 92868
(714) 456-8200

University of California at San Diego Cancer Center**
9500 Gilman Dr., Mail Code 0658
La Jolla, CA 92093-0658
(619) 822-1222
(619) 822-0207

COLORADO
University of Colorado Cancer Center*
4200 East Ninth Avenue
Box E190
Denver, CO 80262
(303) 372-1550

CONNECTICUT
Yale Cancer Center*
Yale University School of Medicine
333 Cedar Street
New Haven, CT 06520-8028
(203) 785-4095

DISTRICT OF COLUMBIA
Lombardi Cancer Center*
Georgetown University Medical Center
3800 Reservoir Road, NW
Washington, DC 20007
(202) 784-4000

FLORIDA
H. Lee Moffitt Cancer Center & Research Institute at the
University of South Florida**
12902 Magnolia Drive
Tampa, FL 33612-9497
(813) 972-4673

HAWAII
Cancer Research Center of Hawaii**
University of Hawai'i
1236 Lauhala Street
Honolulu, HI 96813
(808) 586-3013

◆ ◆

ILLINOIS
Robert H. Lurie Cancer Center*
Northwestern University
Olson Pavilion 8250
710 North Fairbanks Ct.
Chicago, IL 60611-3013
(312) 908-5250

University of Chicago Cancer Research Center*
5841 South Maryland Avenue
Chicago, IL 60637-1470
(888) 824-0200
(773) 702-9200

MARYLAND
The Johns Hopkins Oncology Center*
600 North Wolfe Street
Baltimore, MD 21287-8943
(410) 955-8964

MASSACHUSETTS
Dana-Farber Cancer Institute*
44 Binney Street
Boston, MA 02115
(800) 320-0022
(617) 632-3000

MICHIGAN
Barbara Ann Karmanos Cancer Institute*
Wertz Clinical Cancer Center
4100 John R. Street
Detroit, MI 48201-1379
(800) 527-6266
(888) 527-6266

University of Michigan Comprehensive Cancer Center*
1500 E. Medical Center Drive
Ann Arbor, MI 48109-0843
(800) 865-1125

MINNESOTA
Mayo Clinical Cancer Center**
200 First Street Southwest
Rochester, MN 55905
(507) 284-9589

University of Minnesota Cancer Center**
Box 806
420 Delaware Street, SE
Minneapolis, MN 55455
(612) 624-8484

NEW HAMPSHIRE
Norris Cotton Cancer Center*
Dartmouth-Hitchcock Medical Center
One Medical Center Drive
Lebanon, NH 03756-0001
(603) 650-5527
(800) 639-6918

NEW JERSEY
Cancer Institute of New Jersey**
Robert Wood Johnson Medical School
195 Little Albany Street
New Brunswick, NJ 08901
(732) 235-6777

NEW YORK
Memorial Sloan-Kettering Cancer Center*
1275 York Avenue
New York, NY 10021
(800) 525-2225

◆　◆　◆　◆　◆　◆　◆　◆　◆　◆　◆　◆　◆　◆　◆　◆　◆　◆　◆　◆

Roswell Park Cancer Institute*
Elm and Carlton Streets
Buffalo, NY 14263-0001
(800) 767-9355

Kaplan Comprehensive Cancer Center*
New York University Medical Center
550 First Avenue
New York, NY 10016
(212) 263-6485

Herbert Irving Comprehensive Cancer Center*
Columbia University
Sixth Floor, Room 435
Milstein Hospital Building
177 Fort Washington Avenue
New York, NY 10032
(212) 305-8610

Albert Einstein Comprehensive Cancer Center*
Albert Einstein College of Medicine
300 Morris Park Ave.
Bronx, NY 10461
(718) 430-2302

University of Rochester Cancer Center**
601 Elmwood Avenue, Box 704
Rochester, NY 14642
(716) 275-4911

NORTH CAROLINA
Duke Comprehensive Cancer Center*
Duke University Medical Center
Box 3843
Durham, NC 27710
(919) 684-3377

UNC Lineberger Comprehensive Cancer Center*
University of North Carolina Chapel Hill
School of Medicine, CB-7295
102 West Drive
Chapel Hill, NC 27599-7295
(919) 966-3036
(919) 966-1101

Comprehensive Cancer Center at Wake Forest University*
Baptist Medical Center
Medical Center Boulevard
Winston-Salem, NC 27157-1082
(336) 716-2075

OHIO
Ohio State University Comprehensive Cancer Center*
Arthur G. James Cancer Hospital & Research Institute
300 West 10th Avenue
Columbus, OH 43210-1240
(800) 293-5066

University Hospitals of Cleveland
Ireland Cancer Center*
11100 Euclid Avenue
Cleveland, OH 44106-5065
(800) 641-2422
(216) 844-5432

OREGON
Oregon Health Sciences University**
3181 Southwest Sam Jackson Park Road
Portland, OR 97201-3098
(503) 494-9000

PENNSYLANIA
Fox Chase Cancer Center*
7701 Burholme Avenue
Philadelphia, PA 19111
(215) 728-6900
(888) 369-2427

University of Pennsylvania Cancer Center*
15th Floor, Penn Tower Hotel
3400 Spruce Street
Philadelphia, PA 19104-4383
(800) 383-8722
(215) 662-6364

University of Pittsburgh Cancer Institute*
Information and Referral Service
Suite 206, Iroquois Building
3600 Forbes Avenue
Pittsburgh, PA 15213-3410
(800) 237-4724

Kimmel Cancer Center**
Thomas Jefferson University
Suite 1014
College Building
1025 Walnut Street
Philadelphia, PA 19107
(800) 426-3895
(800) 533-3669

TENNESSEE
St. Jude Children's Research Hospital**
332 North Lauderdale Street
Memphis, TN 38105-0318
(901) 495-3300
(888) 226-4343

Vanderbilt Cancer Center**
Vanderbilt University
649 Medical Research Building II
Nashville, TN 37232-6838
(800) 811-8480
(615) 936-1782

TEXAS
The University of Texas M. D. Anderson Cancer Center*
1515 Holcombe Boulevard
Houston, TX 77030
(800) 392-1611

San Antonio Cancer Institute*
8122 Datapoint Drive
San Antonio, TX 78229-3264
(210) 616-5590

UTAH
Huntsman Cancer Institute**
University of Utah
Room 2100
15 North 2030 East
Salt Lake City, UT 84112-5330
(800) 488-2422
(801) 581-6365

VERMONT
Vermont Cancer Center*
University of Vermont
Medical Alumni Bldg.
Burlington, VT 05405-0068
(802) 656-4414

VIRGINIA
Massey Cancer Center**
Virginia Commonwealth University
P.O. Box 980037
401 College Street
Richmond, VA 23298-0037
(804) 828-0450

Cancer Center at University of Virginia**
P.O. Box 334
Charlottesville, VA 22908
(800) 223-9173
(804) 924-9333

WASHINGTON
Fred Hutchinson Cancer Research Center*
1100 Fairview Avenue North—FM-252
P.O. Box 19024
Seattle, WA 98109-1024
(800) 804-8824
(206) 667-4324

WISCONSIN
University of Wisconsin Comprehensive Cancer Center*
600 Highland Avenue
Madison, WI 53792-0001
(608) 263-8600
(800) 622-8922

◆ ◆ ◆ ◆ ◆ ◆ ◆ ◆ ◆ ◆ ◆ ◆ ◆ ◆ ◆ ◆ ◆ ◆ ◆

BASIC SCIENCE CANCER CENTERS SUPPORTED BY THE NATIONAL CANCER INSTITUTE

The Burnham Institute
La Jolla, California
(619) 455-6480

Armand Hammer Center for Cancer Biology, Salk Institute
La Jolla, California
(619) 453-4100

Purdue Cancer Center,
Purdue University
West Lafayette, Indiana
(765) 494-9129

The Jackson Laboratory
Bar Harbor, Maine
(207) 288-6000

Center for Cancer Research, Massachusetts Institute of Technology
Cambridge, Massachusetts
(617) 253-6422

Eppley Institute, University of Nebraska Medical Center
Omaha, Nebraska
(402) 559-4238

American Health Foundation
New York, New York
(212) 953-1400
(212) 529-0700

Cold Spring Harbor Laboratory
Cold Spring Harbor, New York
(516) 367-8383

Wistar Institute
Philadelphia, Pennsylvania
(215) 898-3926

McArdle Laboratory for Cancer Research, University of Wisconsin
Madison, Wisconsin
(608) 263-8610

THE COMPUTER-FRIENDLY BREAST CANCER SURVIVOR

Online information seekers should visit the NABCO Web site at www.nabco.org. NABCO's site has extensive information, including Fact Sheets, *NABCO News* editions, excerpts of this *Resource List* including the directory of local support groups, and links to numerous other Web sites of interest. Also see the e-mail addresses and Web sites for other resources listed throughout this *List*, and for the national breast cancer organizations.

Good Links. Since breast cancer information on the Web changes rapidly, we recommend the following reputable sites that have good links to other Web sites:

• **Can Search** (National Coalition for Cancer Survivorship) (www.cansearch.org)

• **National Action Plan on Breast Cancer** (www.napbc.org)

• **National Women's Health Information Center** (www.4woman.org)

• **NCI's Cancer Trials** (cancertrials.nci.nih.gov)

• **Oncolink** (cancer.med.upenn.edu)

• **The National Cancer Institute** (cancer.nci.nih.gov)

www.rosieo.warnerbros.com

www.breastdoc.com—Dr. Deborah Axelrod's Web site offers educational information on breast health and cancer as well as breast care resources.

World Resources Institute (www.wri.org)

Journal Searches. Medline is the largest online database, with 3,600 contributing medical journals. Medline has a separate database called Cancerlit. Some public libraries and medical libraries subscribe, and will permit searches, sometimes for a fee. Medline is available at no cost on the Web through HealthGate at www.healthgate.com. You can also use special software such as Grateful Med at igm.nlm.nih.gov. CompuServe and America Online also provide access to Medline.

MAJOR NATIONAL BREAST CANCER ORGANIZATIONS:

NABCO, 9 East 37th Street, 10th Floor, New York, NY 10016, (888) 80-NABCO.

The National Breast Cancer Coalition, 1707 L Street, NW, Suite 1060, Washington, DC 20036, (202) 296-7477.

American Cancer Society, (800) ACS-2345.

The Susan G. Komen Breast Cancer Foundation and Race for the Cure®, 5005 LBJ Freeway, Suite 370, Dallas, TX 75244, (972) 855-1600 or (800) I'M AWARE.

Y-ME National Breast Cancer Organization, 212 W. Van Buren Street, Fifth Floor, Chicago, IL 60607, (800) 221-2141.

National Action Plan on Breast Cancer, www.napbc.org/napbc/volguide.htm.

Cancer Care, www.cancercare.org.

The Breast Cancer Fund, 282 Second St, 2nd Floor, San Francisco, CA 94105, (800) 487-0492, www.breastcancerfund.org.

◆   ◆   ◆   ◆   ◆   ◆   ◆   ◆   ◆   ◆   ◆   ◆   ◆   ◆   ◆   ◆   ◆

U.S. ORGANIZATIONS AND PROJECTS
ON THE HEALTH OF WOMEN OF COLOR

(COURTESY OF MICHELLE JOHNSON, M.D., MPH, CRESHELL NASH, M.D., MPH, NANCY TORRES, M.D., MPH, AND JOAN REEDE, M.D., MPH)

The National Asian Women's Health Organization, a nonprofit, community-based organization established in 1993, has researched the impact of tobacco on Asian-American women to inform policy; past research has focused on reproductive and sexual health.

National Asian Women's Health Organization
250 Montgomery St, Suite 410
San Francisco, CA 94104
415-989-9747; nawho@nawho.org

Asians and Pacific Islanders for Reproductive Health is the nation's first community-based nonprofit organization devoted to promoting quality reproductive health care for Asians and Pacific Islanders.

Asians and Pacific Islanders
for Reproductive Health
310 Eighth St, Suite 100
Oakland, CA 94607
510-268-8988; apirh@apirh.org

The National Latina Health Organization's purpose is "to advocate, educate, and support the right of Latinas to preventive health practices, early detection of health threats, and a full range of quality health interventions and care."

National Latina Health Organization
PO Box 7567
Oakland, CA 94601
510-534-1362
http://latino.sscnet.ucla.edu/women/nlho

The National Council of Negro Women has a long history of concern for the health of women of color. Its Reproductive Health Information Agenda has been used to increase public awareness; recent efforts have targeted sexually transmitted diseases and increased funding for research on the health of women of color.

National Council of Negro Women
633 Pennsylvania Ave, NW
Washington, DC 20004
202-737-0120; info@ncw.com

Established in 1971, the **National Black Nurses Association** advocates for the health care needs of African Americans. Its Women's Health Research Program develops knowledge on African American biopsychosocial characteristics and their relationship to menopause and menstrual health.

National Black Nurses Association
1511 K St, NW, Suite 415
Washington, DC 20005
202-393-6870; www.nbna.org

The **National Black Women's Health Project** advocates for recruiting women of color into clinical trials and for women of color in key administrative positions in health research. Current research includes access, welfare reform, and insurance, and their impact on women of color.

The National Black Women's Health Project
1211 Connecticut Ave, NW, Suite 310
Washington, DC 20036
202-835-0117; nbwhpdc@aol.com

The **Asian and Pacific Islander American Health Forum** has established a Women's Health Information Network. It researched the effects of Medi-Cal on API women to make recommendations for consumers, managed care organizations, and the California Department of Health Services.

Asian and Pacific Islander
American Health Forum
942 Market St, Suite 200
San Francisco, CA 94102
415-954-9959; marnelle@apiahf.org

Created in 1996 to ensure that California health policies are responsive to the needs of Latinas, the **Latina Health Project** gathers primary and secondary data on Latina health indicators, monitors and analyzes state and national policies, and meets with policy makers.

Latina Health Project
1535 Mission St
San Francisco, CA 94103
415-431-7430
http://www.lchc.org/lhppind.htm

The National Coalition of Hispanic Health and Human Services is involved in research on the disproportionate impact of diabetes on Hispanic women as well as investigating reasons for their use of preventive services.

National Coalition of Hispanic Health and Human Services
1501 16th St, NW
Washington, DC 20036
202-387-5000; info@cossmho.org

The National Medical Association has identified women's health as one of its public health objectives; the African American Women's Health Promotion in Breast and Cervical Cancer seeks to better understand black women's acceptance of and compliance with screening recommendations.

National Medical Association
1012 Tenth St, NW
Washington, DC 20001
202-347-1895; www.NMAnet.org

Current priorities of **The Society for the Advancement of Women's Health Research** include fostering the recruitment and retention of minorities and women in clinical trials.

Society for the Advancement of Women's Health Research
1828 L St, NW, Suite 625
Washington, DC 20036
202-223-8224
information@womens-health.org

BREAST CANCER RESOURCES

I	M	K	U	I	A	C	D	V	A	O	I	G	Q	N	N
E	R	Y	W	Z	A	S	D	Q	D	I	M	K	V	M	N
S	F	C	X	R	Q	U	H	O	S	P	I	T	A	L	S
E	G	A	V	F	H	P	A	O	U	O	S	E	H	C	R
N	Z	C	Q	V	W	P	N	R	Y	Q	S	M	S	N	O
I	W	O	J	O	G	O	D	N	W	T	E	Z	A	S	V
L	N	V	V	O	L	R	S	B	O	E	S	Z	B	R	I
T	E	D	U	C	A	T	I	O	N	L	R	R	H	E	V
O	R	A	N	V	U	G	T	E	C	W	U	R	R	N	R
H	D	F	U	N	D	R	A	I	S	I	N	G	Y	T	U
W	L	I	T	Y	O	O	I	H	D	S	E	D	H	R	S
D	I	M	X	M	C	U	B	L	L	W	R	T	Y	A	K
W	H	C	Z	N	T	P	G	N	I	P	O	C	I	P	F
U	C	L	D	I	O	S	C	V	L	C	Q	Q	D	E	I
C	A	N	C	E	R	C	E	N	T	E	R	S	Z	N	S
K	S	P	X	T	S	H	D	C	G	S	M	J	L	Y	Z

Find and circle the following words:

ADVOCACY	EDUCATION	PARTNERS
CANCER CENTERS	FUND-RAISING	SOCIETIES
CHILDREN	HOSPITALS	SUPPORT GROUPS
COPING	HOTLINES	SURVIVORS
DOCTORS	NURSES	

TAKE TWO

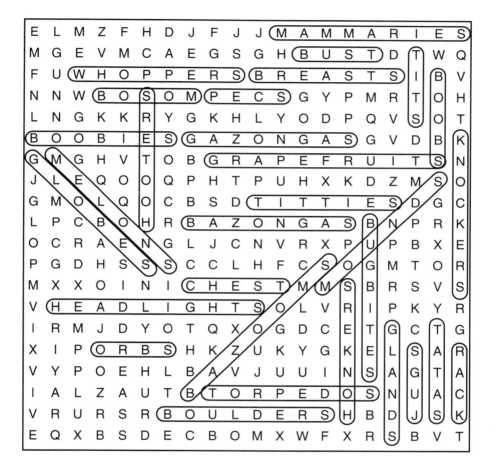

E	L	M	Z	F	H	D	J	F	J	J	M	A	M	M	A	R	I	E	S
M	G	E	V	M	C	A	E	G	S	G	H	B	U	S	T	D	T	W	Q
F	U	W	H	O	P	P	E	R	S	B	R	E	A	S	T	S	I	B	V
N	N	W	B	O	S	O	M	P	E	C	S	G	Y	P	M	R	T	O	H
L	N	G	K	K	R	Y	G	K	H	L	Y	O	D	P	Q	V	S	O	T
B	O	O	B	I	E	S	G	A	Z	O	N	G	A	S	G	V	D	B	K
G	M	G	H	V	T	O	B	G	R	A	P	E	F	R	U	I	T	S	N
J	L	E	Q	O	O	Q	P	H	T	P	U	H	X	K	D	Z	M	S	O
G	M	O	L	Q	O	C	B	S	D	T	I	T	T	I	E	S	D	G	C
L	P	C	B	O	H	R	B	A	Z	O	N	G	A	S	B	N	P	R	K
O	C	R	A	E	N	G	L	J	C	N	V	R	X	P	U	P	B	X	E
P	G	D	H	S	S	S	C	C	L	H	F	C	S	O	G	M	T	O	R
M	X	X	O	I	N	I	C	H	E	S	T	M	M	S	B	R	S	V	S
V	H	E	A	D	L	I	G	H	T	S	O	L	V	R	I	P	K	Y	R
I	R	M	J	D	Y	O	T	Q	X	O	G	D	C	E	T	G	C	T	G
X	I	P	O	R	B	S	H	K	Z	U	K	Y	G	K	E	L	S	A	R
V	Y	P	O	E	H	L	B	A	V	J	U	U	I	N	S	A	G	T	A
I	A	L	Z	A	U	T	B	T	O	R	P	E	D	O	S	N	U	A	C
V	R	U	R	S	R	B	O	U	L	D	E	R	S	H	B	D	J	S	K
E	Q	X	B	S	D	E	C	B	O	M	X	W	F	X	R	S	B	V	T

BAZONGAS	BREASTS	GLOBES	KNOCKERS	RACK
BAZOOMS	BUGBITES	GRAPEFRUITS	MAMMARIES	TATAS
BOOBIES	BUST	HEADLIGHTS	MELONS	TITS
BOOBS	CHEST	HONKERS	MOUNDS	TITTIES
BOSOM	GAZONGAS	HOOTERS	ORBS	TORPEDOS
BOULDERS	GLANDS	JUGS	PECS	WHOPPERS

KEEPING ABREAST OF THE PROBLEM

```
Y  A  C  K  C  K  F  P  W  X  K  O  C  T  B  Y
C  T  Q  N  M  D  X  X  O  W  Y  K  X  R  J  S
R  N  O  W  W  R  R  K  A  L  N  A  P  A  J  A
C  L  S  N  E  G  O  R  T  S  E  O  T  Y  H  P
F  Y  S  R  C  B  W  E  J  J  U  G  H  A  T  K
D  A  P  N  E  G  O  R  T  S  E  G  X  Y  W  O
I  N  B  P  L  O  N  G  I  S  L  A  N  D  L  L
R  W  V  T  H  S  W  L  A  V  F  G  O  L  H  V
N  U  O  L  U  J  I  R  M  W  F  R  C  J  A  C
R  T  A  F  Y  R  A  T  E  I  D  U  H  G  L  K
Q  A  R  S  L  F  F  I  N  L  A  N  D  I  N  W
O  S  E  D  I  C  I  T  S  E  P  F  W  N  D  O
K  K  M  E  F  N  K  M  Z  X  Q  G  I  E  I  M
O  T  Z  W  T  O  E  Y  L  N  K  U  F  B  W  E
Z  Z  X  H  E  I  G  O  U  J  W  Y  O  T  E  N
R  M  O  M  E  N  J  K  I  O  P  P  Y  O  S  R
```

DIETARY FAT	JAPAN	PHYTOESTROGENS
ESTROGEN	LONG ISLAND	SOY
FIBER	MEN	WOMEN
FINLAND	PESTICIDES	

BREAST HEALTH AND ANATOMY

```
Y  S  F  F  Q  V  P  P  S  V  J  T  H  P
R  W (D  I  S  C  H  A  R  G  E) A  S  J
K  O  O  G  S  X  L  E  I  H  X  F  J  C
S  R  Q  R  G  V  E  O  W  W  D  S  H  N
(D  U  C  T  S) V  P (N  U  R  S  I  N  G)
J  Q  H  O  M  Q  R  L  T  S  T  D  Q  U
(S  E  L  F  E  X  A  M) K  S  W  F  G  Y
(N  I  P  P  L  E) W  T  A  L  D  F  Z  K
R  I  B  J  U  W  B  E  C  O  X  P  N  L
(A  R  E  O  L  A) R  L  T  B  E  H  M  R
N  X  T  S  J  B  W  U  W  U  X  U  J  M
R  T  C  T  D  S  M  M  Y  L  W  Z  T  U
M  A  R  M  I  Z  Z  P  S  E  O  W  B  O
I  N  L  Z  H  G  E  J  Y  S  O  K  Q  R
```

AREOLA   DUCTS   LUMP   NURSING
BREAST   LOBULES   NIPPLE   SELF-EXAM
DISCHARGE

THE BIG SQUEEZE

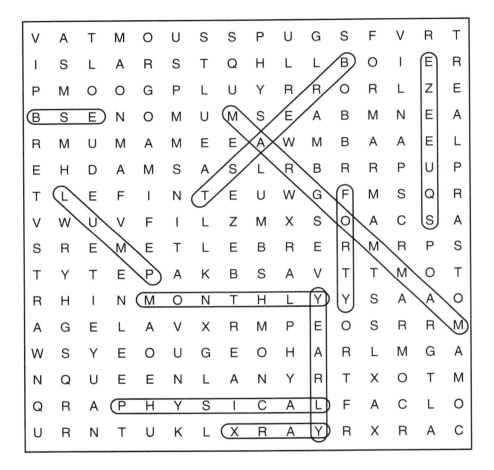

BSE	PHYSICAL	MAMMOGRAM
MONTHLY	SQUEEZE	FORTY
X RAY	BREAST	
YEARLY	LUMP	

BREAST CANCER RISK—AND RISK REDUCTION

```
N  U  T  Z  B  Z  N  G  S  O  Y  F  R  L  J  A
Y  W  J  J  N  W  S  F  B  W  N  T  A  N  H  L
H  F  I  B  E  R  Q  Y  D  Y  E  D  D  Z  C  R
Q  L  S  R  C  R  D  C  Q  O  G  P  I  X  S  Y
Y  E  A  Q  S  X  D  H  D  B  O  U  A  R  B  T
D  S  C  I  T  E  N  E  G  D  R  W  T  M  T  T
P  U  A  Y  M  B  D  V  N  T  T  Z  I  Z  H  E
Y  P  R  E  G  N  A  N  C  Y  S  S  O  W  E  Z
F  R  K  Q  W  Q  Q  P  I  F  E  Y  N  W  P  R
F  Q  W  B  U  Q  N  T  J  Y  J  R  B  P  I  B
N  G  N  I  D  E  E  F  T  S  A  E  R  B  L  F
F  Y  A  E  Y  Q  G  P  S  A  L  C  O  R  L  I
S  H  J  W  M  Z  I  A  V  L  S  N  H  W  G  C
Q  Q  U  F  H  U  C  Y  S  T  X  J  A  F  B  V
Y  A  V  K  P  A  O  B  E  S  I  T  Y  U  W  X
H  H  W  Q  Z  L  O  H  O  C  L  A  J  E  F  O
```

ALCOHOL
BREAST-FEEDING
DES
ESTROGEN

FIBER
GENETICS
OBESITY

PREGNANCY
RADIATION
THE PILL

DIAGNOSIS

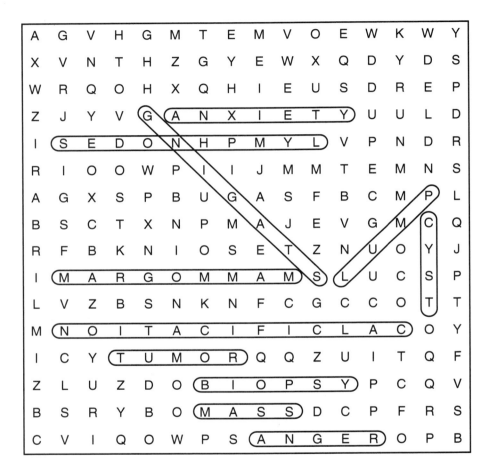

ANGER
ANXIETY
BIOPSY
CALCIFICATION

CYST
LUMP
LYMPH NODES
MAMMOGRAM

MASS
STAGING
TUMOR

TREATMENT

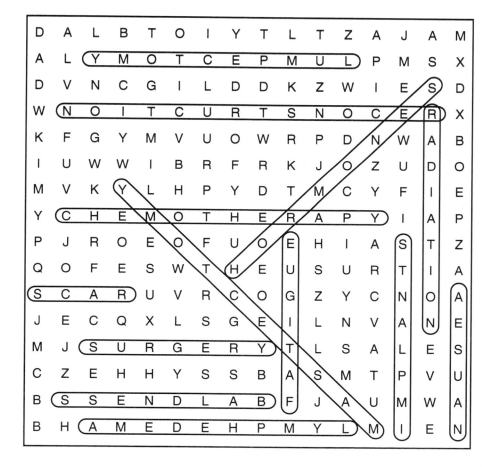

D	A	L	B	T	O	I	Y	T	L	T	Z	A	J	A	M
A	L	Y	M	O	T	C	E	P	M	U	L	P	M	S	X
D	V	N	C	G	I	L	D	D	K	Z	W	I	E	S	D
W	N	O	I	T	C	U	R	T	S	N	O	C	E	R	X
K	F	G	Y	M	V	U	O	W	R	P	D	N	W	A	B
I	U	W	W	I	B	R	F	R	K	J	O	Z	U	D	O
M	V	K	Y	L	H	P	Y	D	T	M	C	Y	F	I	E
Y	C	H	E	M	O	T	H	E	R	A	P	Y	I	A	P
P	J	R	O	E	F	U	O	E	H	I	A	S	T	Z
Q	O	F	E	S	W	T	H	E	U	S	U	R	T	I	A
S	C	A	R	U	V	R	C	O	G	Z	Y	C	N	O	A
J	E	C	Q	X	L	S	G	E	I	L	N	V	A	N	E
M	J	S	U	R	G	E	R	Y	T	L	S	A	L	E	S
C	Z	E	H	H	Y	S	S	B	A	S	M	T	P	V	U
B	S	S	E	N	D	L	A	B	F	J	A	U	M	W	A
B	H	A	M	E	D	E	H	P	M	Y	L	M	I	E	N

BALDNESS   LUMPECTOMY   RADIATION
CHEMOTHERAPY   LYMPHEDEMA   RECONSTRUCTION
FATIGUE   MASTECTOMY   SCAR
HORMONES   NAUSEA   SURGERY
IMPLANTS

AFTERCARE

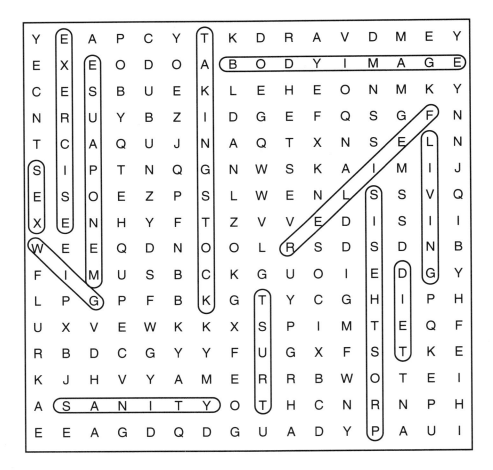

Y	E	A	P	C	Y	T	K	D	R	A	V	D	M	E	Y
E	X	E	O	D	O	A	B	O	D	Y	I	M	A	G	E
C	E	S	B	U	E	K	L	E	H	E	O	N	M	K	Y
N	R	U	Y	B	Z	I	D	G	E	F	Q	S	G	F	N
T	C	A	Q	U	J	N	A	Q	T	X	N	S	E	L	N
S	I	P	T	N	Q	G	N	W	S	K	A	I	M	I	J
E	S	O	E	Z	P	S	L	W	E	N	L	S	S	V	Q
X	E	N	H	Y	F	T	Z	V	V	E	D	I	S	I	I
W	E	E	Q	D	N	O	O	L	R	S	D	S	D	N	B
F	I	M	U	S	B	C	K	G	U	O	I	E	D	G	Y
L	P	G	P	F	B	K	G	T	Y	C	G	H	I	P	H
U	X	V	E	W	K	K	X	S	P	I	M	T	E	Q	F
R	B	D	C	G	Y	Y	F	U	G	X	F	S	T	K	E
K	J	H	V	Y	A	M	E	R	R	B	W	O	T	E	I
A	S	A	N	I	T	Y	O	T	H	C	N	R	N	P	H
E	E	A	G	D	Q	D	G	U	A	D	Y	P	A	U	I

BODY IMAGE	MENOPAUSE	SEX
DIET	PROSTHESIS	TAKING STOCK
EXERCISE	RELIEF	TRUST
LIVING	SANITY	WIG

BREAST CANCER SURVIVORS

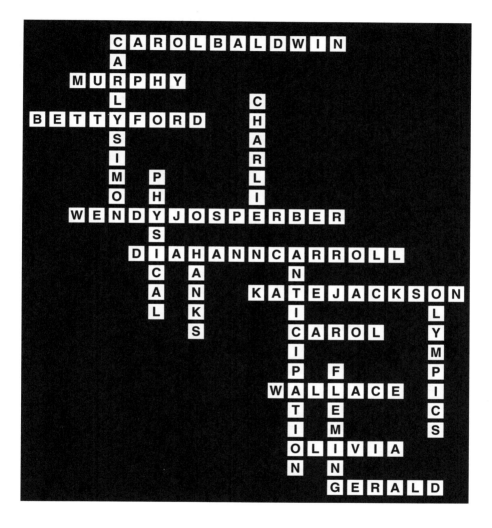

CAROL BALDWIN
CARLYSIMON
MURPHY
BETTY FORD
CHARLIE
WENDYJOSPERBER
PHYSICAL
DIAHANN CARROLL
DICAL
CALS
ANKS
KATE JACKSON
ANTICIPATION
CAROL
OLYMPICS
WALLACE
FLEMING
OLIVIA
GERALD

BREAST CANCER—THE FUTURE

```
I  B  S  Z  T  I  D  K  J  D  G  I  S  P  I  A  J  T  W  E
Z  N  N  S  J  G  T  J  Z  Q  S  I  O  Z  F  I  V  W (S) I
R  K  D  S  E  M  G  R  D  I  A  W  V  N  H  H  N  B  E  M
K  M  H  Q  X  S  H  D  D  S  G  Y  W (C) A  A  O  R  N  S
D  Z (G  E  N  E  S) V  U  P  C  G  M  H  V  N  D  T  I  Z
F  K  I  I  S  Z  K  X  X  D  N  R  W  E  L  E  V  G  C  U
O  I  Q  B  F  F  E  X  M  A  M  N  H  M  R  U  M  I  C  G
X  R  X  P  H  S  J  Z  Y  P  X  E  E  O  L  T  P  M  A  G
L  C  G  C  P  M  K  J  I  E  H  D  E  P  A  K  O  X  V  N
V  P  B  V  C  V  I  N  S  A  U  J  D  R  P  F  V  G  B  V
N  K  V  E  C  K  V  K  X  R  L  N  E  E  B  Y  E  J  Y  H
F  H  W  M  C  B  J  U  F  M  X  P  G  V  S  U  W  M  P  P
P  Y  F  T  U  V  S  C  M  G  W  P  B  E  B  O  B  K  Y  H
J  V  A  P  N  M  L  A  R  Z  Y  K  O  N  H  R  R  N  A  Q
X  P  P  E  W  Q  V  K  M  L  K  E  G  T  B  N  Z  V  K  H
(M  O  N  O  C  L  O  N  A  L  A  N  T  I  B  O  D  I  E  S)
V  N  Q  G  K  M  T  N  B  M  Q  J  S  O  J  K  X  S  I  U
C  U  N  Z  V  L  M  D  N  R  M  N  N  N  G  A  Y  I  B  R
B  N  S  W  A  A  B  M  A  D  J  K  N  K  Y  N  X  H  X  L
J  T  V  X  W  B  G  B  V  Q  C  G  P  V  E  C  S  Y  U  I
```

CHEMOPREVENTION
GENES

MONOCLONAL ANTIBODIES
VACCINES

BREAST CANCER RESOURCES

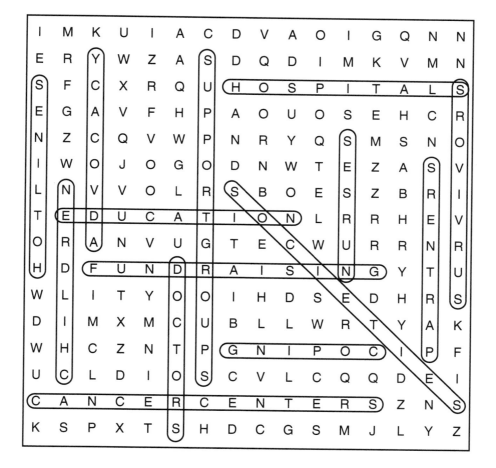

```
I  M  K  U  I  A  C  D  V  A  O  I  G  Q  N  N
E  R  Y  W  Z  A  S  D  Q  D  I  M  K  V  M  N
S  F  C  X  R  Q  U  H  O  S  P  I  T  A  L  S
E  G  A  V  F  H  P  A  O  U  O  S  E  H  C  R
N  Z  C  Q  V  W  P  N  R  Y  Q  S  M  S  N  O
I  W  O  J  O  G  O  D  N  W  T  E  Z  A  S  V
L  N  V  V  O  L  R  S  B  O  E  S  Z  B  R  I
T  E  D  U  C  A  T  I  O  N  L  R  R  H  E  V
O  R  A  N  V  U  G  T  E  C  W  U  R  R  N  R
H  D  F  U  N  D  R  A  I  S  I  N  G  Y  T  U
W  L  I  T  Y  O  O  I  H  D  S  E  D  H  R  S
D  I  M  X  M  C  U  B  L  L  W  R  T  Y  A  K
W  H  C  Z  N  T  P  G  N  I  P  O  C  I  P  F
U  C  L  D  I  O  S  C  V  L  C  Q  Q  D  E  I
C  A  N  C  E  R  C  E  N  T  E  R  S  Z  N  S
K  S  P  X  T  S  H  D  C  G  S  M  J  L  Y  Z
```

ADVOCACY

CANCER CENTERS

CHILDREN

COPING

DOCTORS

EDUCATION

FUND-RAISING

HOSPITALS

HOTLINES

NURSES

PARTNERS

SOCIETIES

SUPPORT GROUPS

SURVIVORS

ABOUT THE AUTHORS

A board-certified surgeon who specializes in breast diseases and breast cancer, DR. DEBORAH AXELROD, formerly physician in charge of the Louis Venet, M.D., Comprehensive Breast Service at Beth Israel Medical Center, New York City, is chief of the Breast Center at St. Vincent's Comprehensive Cancer Center and associate professor of surgery at New York Medical College. A fellow of the American College of Surgeons, Dr. Axelrod completed a surgical oncology research fellowship at Memorial Sloan-Kettering Cancer Center. She is widely published in her field, and has been in practice since 1988.

A television producer and journalist specializing in health issues, TRACY CHUTORIAN SEMLER is the author of *All About Eve: The Complete Guide to Women's Health and Well-Being* and the forthcoming *The Fit Brain*. She wrote and produced the award-winning five-part series "American Woman" for *CBS Morning News*, and is cocreator of the www.MDWomens Health.com Web site.